T0160892

Cancer on Two Wheels is the remarkable journey of a man's love for the Lord deepening even in the worst of times. Chris Haga takes us along with him on the spiritual ride of his life that will inspire you to cling to God every day. For those questioning God's purpose for trials in their life, this legacy of hope and faith is a must read.

—Dr. Robert Jeffress
Senior Pastor
First Baptist Church, Dallas
Bible Teacher, Pathway to Victory

Perhaps the most compelling attribute of *Cancer on Two Wheels* is that the author allows us into some of his most personal thoughts and feelings—something very difficult for most to share. Although we will never be able to understand the depth of his experience, he nonetheless weaves his thoughts into analogies of God's love and grace like a pastor from the pulpit. Chris Haga reminds us of the promise that God continues to walk hand in hand with us and is already preparing the path for each of us long before we take those steps.

—Gregg Groves

Chris Haga's writing is amazing. Just the right tone, always the right words, and so wonderfully insightful and inspirational.

—Robin McGee

The author amazes me by the way he expresses himself in such a talented manner and how he witnesses in the midst of his own struggles.

—Matt Middleton

I have gained a new and fresh perspective of the Lord and how He works in our lives. I have been encouraged and reminded of God's love through *Cancer on Two Wheels*. The author has a way of putting his feelings and spiritual battles into written words that transcend time and cancer. Through his encouraging writings, God speaks to me. I don't have cancer, but I have other trials, and I know that God is with me through all of them. I know that He cares. Thank you for reminding me of that.

—Amy Smith

I am moved and inspired by the author's courage, but most importantly by his witness and faith. Even during his bad days, he runs to his faith and not away from it. The light of Christ shines brightly through Chris Haga's writings.

—Curry Vogelsang

God has worked in my heart through reading *Cancer on Two Wheels*. He has faithfully used Chris Haga to encourage me and give me wisdom. Light in darkness. Powerful truth. Faithful witness.

—Mary Havey

CANCER ON TWO WHEELS

A Spiritual Journey with Stage IV Lung Cancer

CHRIS HAGA

Carpenter's Son Publishing

Cancer on Two Wheels

©2018 by Chris and DeLayne Haga

All rights reserved. No part of this book may be reproduced or transmitted in any form or by any means, electronic or mechanical, including photocopying, recording, or by any information storage and retrieval system, without permission in writing from the copyright owner.

Published by Carpenter's Son Publishing, Franklin, Tennessee

Published in association with Larry Carpenter
of Christian Book Services, LLC
www.christianbookservices.com

Published in association with Roaring Lambs Publishing, Dallas, Texas

Scripture taken from the NEW AMERICAN STANDARD BIBLE®, Copyright © 1960,1962,1963,1968,1971,1972,1973,1975,1977,1995 by The Lockman Foundation. Used by permission.

Cover Image used by permission of alphaspirit at 123RF.com.

Senior Editor: Tammy Kling

Assistant Editor: Tiarra Tompkins

Copy Editors: Christy Callahan, Lee Ann Bandy, and Kristi Brashier

Cover and Interior Design: Suzanne Lawing

Printed in the United States of America

ISBN 978-1-946889-62-1

*To our sons, Chad and Shane, the best
wingmen a father could have asked for*

*To all our prayer warriors for hoisting us on your
shoulders while you were on your knees in prayer*

To God—may Your name be glorified

CONTENTS

Foreword 13

Diagnosis 15

Questions 17

Wingmen 19

The Sycamore Tree 23

Eye of the Storm 25

Pepper 27

Changes 29

Finding the Right Gear 31

Blessed Assurance 33

Friends 36

Hope: Part 1 38

Hope: Part 2 41

Hope: Part 3 43

Hope: Part 4 45

Hope: Part 5 47

Hope: Part 6 49

Stinkin' Thinkin' 51

I'll Tell You a Secret 53

Area Fifty-One 55

Rear-View Mirrors 58

It's a Wonderful Life 60

My Psalm 62

The Process 63

Old Stories: Noah 66

The Greatest Man I Have Ever Known 68

In the Cloud 72

A Dad, a Son, and His Bikes 74

Prayers 77

A Life Sentence 79

More Than I Can Handle 81

Sin and Love Held Him There 83

Right People, Right Place, Right Time 85

Chasing Dreams 87

Wet Feet 89

Limits 91

Things Cancer Has Taught Me 93

The Wind at My Back 95

One More Hill 97

Doubts 99

Standing on the Pedals 100

Purpose: Part 1 102

What a View 104

B-52 106

A Broken Vessel 108

The Pathway Back 110

Wrestling with Satan 112

The Next Step 114

The Potter and His Clay. 115

Twenty-One. 116

Purpose: Part 2 118

Uncertainty 120

Lessons from a Dead Battery 121

No Smell of Fire 123

Pruning 125

Deep Roots 126

Picking Up Bread Crumbs 128

Mountaintops and Valleys. 130

Grapefruit 131

Armor Fitting 133

Put Me In, Coach 135

When Dreams Intersect. 137

God and Pickup Trucks. 143

No Evidence of Disease 146

Tough as Leather 148

The Best 150

Learning to Fly 152

Not Letting Go 154

Thirty Years 156

Unknown Land. 160

A Collection of Randomness 162

Cups 166

Unbelief 167

Living Psalm 13 169

Vacation! 171

Made It to Five Years 172

Have I Been a Fool? 175

A Good Ride 177

Do Not Worry 179

The Last Word 181

Afterword: Paying Homage 183

Appendix: Lung Cancer Statistics and Symptoms . . . 185

About the Author 189

FOREWORD

By DeLayne Haga

In 2010, the love of my life was diagnosed with stage IV lung cancer that had metastasized to his brain. I was stunned—*he had never smoked.*

The mass in my husband's lung almost tripled in size within three months of his diagnosis to 13 centimeters—almost half the length of a ruler—before we found a successful regimen to shrink the cancer. The doctor originally gave Chris a prognosis of six months. Instead, he lived six *years.* Because he was officially declared to have "no evidence of disease" on three separate occasions, I still refer to him as "My Miracle Man." I witnessed God's glory multiple times.

Chris was riding his bike eighty miles a week when diagnosed. Amazingly, he was able to continue riding his bicycle for several years, even with a collapsed lung.

My husband chronicled his spiritual journey in a blog. Many suggested he turn it into a book because of his gifted, inspirational writings. They appreciated his transparency, as he didn't portray the cancer journey as a bed of roses, and others with cancer could relate to his experience. There were some great times during the battle as well as less than desirable moments. It was obvious when he was struggling and losing hope for survival—especially the third month—as you'll read in "Hope: Part 1." He never posted parts 2–6, thinking they were too negative. I recently came across them in his journal and decided to publish them. Even in deep despair, his continued faith was inspiring. Though his hope in the doctors and medicine faltered, Chris's love for the Lord and his trust in Him never wavered.

My husband wrote about his spiritual insights and topics that were special to him as he realized what—and who—was most important in his life. You'll read about his close relationship with our sons. He tells how his earthly father's life shaped his own. But this isn't a story about a man adoring his children or his earthly father. It's the picture of a man worshiping his heavenly Father even when he didn't feel worshipful.

Chris portrays that it is normal and even acceptable to have doubts and to question God—God expects it. Facing a trial is an opportunity to explore your beliefs and to grow your faith. My husband realized that faith without trials requires no faith at all. Is your faith built on sand that will wash away easily—or rather on solid rock that will withstand the storms in your life?

As you read, please take time to reflect on your own memories. Count your blessings. Let those you love and hold dear to your heart know it. What do you want your legacy to be?

Chris struggled and sought to understand the purpose in having lung cancer. He desperately wanted something good to come from his experience that would help others, but writing a book was never on his radar. I chose to publish his journal to honor his memory as well as to fulfill God's purpose and Chris's desire to glorify Him through his journey of faith.

This book seeks to proclaim how God worked through my husband's life and is still working beyond his death as Chris's spirit lives on. This is his legacy.

I will not die, but live, and tell of the works of the LORD.
—PSALM 118:17

DIAGNOSIS

July 31, 2010

It became official at 3:30 p.m. on July 30. I have lung cancer. Those are two words I never thought I'd hear a doctor tell me.

One question that several people have already asked is, "How did this start?" In April, I was on a bike ride and was headed back home when I got a tickle in my throat and a cough. I didn't think much of it and chalked it up to allergies. The cough steadily got worse over the next few weeks. Then in early May, I had a bad coughing episode at work. I went to the doctor, and he diagnosed it as an upper respiratory infection and put me on an antibiotic for a week. I started feeling better over the next week, but the cough stayed.

DeLayne (my wife) and I took her mom to Atlanta to see her family in mid-May. I felt good but still had the cough. After we returned to Dallas, the cough came back with a vengeance, so I visited my family doctor. He ordered a set of chest x-rays and diagnosed me with pneumonia. I was prescribed another round of antibiotics and was told to come back in ten days so he could check to see if the pneumonia was gone. At my follow-up, he said my lungs were clear, even though I still had my cough. "That's normal for pneumonia," he said.

Over the next three weeks, I continued to ride and noticed that when I rode, my airway opened up, and I could breathe much better. On the morning of July 5, I got up and went for an early-morning ride. I rode almost twenty miles and felt great. Dare I say, I felt fast. This was, without a doubt, the best I'd felt in two months, and I thought that I was finally getting over this stuff.

Later that same morning, I went for my follow-up x-rays and doctor appointment. I about went into shock when he came in and told me that not only did I still have pneumonia, but it was worse. He provided me a pulmonologist's name and said, "See him as soon as you can."

The month of July has been spent seeing either the pulmonologist or going to the hospital for CT scans and biopsies. The last biopsy confirmed I have non-small cell adenocarcinoma in my right lung. At this point, I'm not a good candidate for surgery because of where and how the tumor has grown. We'll now start our search for treatment options.

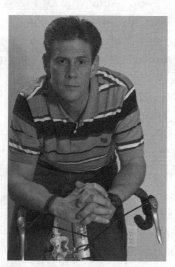

This photograph is of me the day I learned of my cancer diagnosis. The bike I'm on is my road bike. I started riding a few years ago after the boys started riding and racing. I thought I'd go riding with the boys. That didn't last long. The goal finally came to just trying to keep them in sight. So far, the doctors are telling me to keep riding as long as I feel like it.

The morning after getting the diagnosis, I went for a ride. I made sure to ride a little farther than usual. I figured if I could ride just a little beyond the usual distance, it would be a small triumph over the cancer. After the last month, I'll take victories where I can.

I promise to keep this as lighthearted as possible. I'll try not to preach, but God is already opening my eyes to many things, so be prepared.

QUESTIONS

August 2, 2010

I'm learning what every cancer patient has to learn to deal with—the never-ending questions. There are questions from doctors, nurses, friends, and family. The worst ones are the questions from yourself. These are the ones that can keep you awake at night and defeat sleeping aids. So, in the interest of a better night's rest, I'll try to deal with a few of them here.

Why me?

According to the doctor, I'm just one of that small fraction of people who have zero risk factors and still get lung cancer. With my dad having three different cancers and my sister being a breast cancer survivor, maybe it's genetic. For all the people who think I'm a little off, now you know. I might be genetically modified.

In all seriousness, the question just might as well be, *Why not me?* I don't think there's anything so special about me that should guarantee I wouldn't get cancer. I might as well have this as anyone else, and, as of yet, God hasn't chosen to show me His complete plan. I'll take this one day, one step at a time.

Although I accept there's not an answer to this question, and I try not to dwell on it, I'll confess that Sunday evening I did have a real moment. DeLayne, Shane (our younger son), and I decided to run out and get a sandwich. As we walked up to the restaurant, I noticed a guy who had to be fifty to one hundred pounds overweight and smoking a cigarette. The thought popped into my head, *And I'm the guy with lung cancer.*

Should I be mad at God?

No, I don't think so. If I should be mad at anybody, I would go with Adam and Eve. God placed Adam and Eve in the perfect world. Unfortunately, He gave them free will, and they messed it up. As a result, there are bad things in this world. Thankfully, God gave His one and only Son as a way to redemption and eternal life for the rest of us. I can't imagine going through this mess without the knowledge that eventually my home is in heaven.

Will I be healed?

I sincerely believe that I will be. Some of you may think I'm totally off of my rocker with this one, but this actually did happen. It was the Sunday after getting the CT results that identified two tumors in my right lung. Shane and I walked into the sanctuary at church and sat down. I was looking through the order of service and scanned down to the day's message title, "Healed of a Lengthy Affliction." Out of nowhere, I heard a voice say, *It will be a long, hard battle, but you will be healed.* It wasn't a loud, booming voice. I guess I'd call it that still, small voice we all want to hear.

Imagine my surprise today when the pulmonologist said to me, "The bottom line is that you have lung cancer. You're in for a long, hard battle."

Coincidence?

I don't think so.

WINGMEN

August 7, 2010

The term "wingman" was first used in World War I. The U.S. Army Air Corps realized that more of their pilots returned when two or more planes flew together. Your wingman was the pilot who flew just off your wing tip to help cover you from attacks.

One night when I couldn't sleep, I began reviewing the last few years in my mind and some of the bike rides I've been on. I realize the rides that I remember most are the ones I've been on with my sons, Chad and Shane. We've had a lot of fun and probably more than our share of laughs, but I always feel a bit younger and a bit spunkier when I ride with them. We each get our share of barbs in and try to watch out for road hazards. Usually, by the time I reach a hazard, I've had two warnings.

They usually offer me encouragement like this:

"Hurry up, old man."

"Try and keep up at least until we're out of the neighborhood."

"You want me to push you up this hill?"

Here are some of my favorite bike riding stories:

We got up early one morning and decided to take a ride out to Lake Lavon. The ride is about thirty-five miles roundtrip and on two-lane country roads. This particular morning, Chad

had decided to ride his "fixie," which is a fixed-gear bike that can't coast. (If the wheels are spinning, so are your legs. To slow down, you have to slow the spinning of the pedals.)

We were headed downhill on one of the back roads, and Chad was in the lead about twenty yards in front. I was in my usual position, the rear. Suddenly, out of the left ditch pops a skunk and starts running across the road. I hit the brakes and start yelling at Chad to watch the skunk. He finally sees it about five feet from him and locks up his legs, putting his bike in to a skid. Since we escaped unscathed, it was funny. The three of us had a good laugh.

When I first got my road bike and was learning to ride with my feet clipped to the pedals, we went for a quick ride. The wind was really blowing that day out of the south. It took all I had to stay upright. As we were approaching an intersection, our light turned red. I was leaning hard into a crosswind, trying to stop and get unclipped all at the same time. Obviously, it was too much for my mind to handle. I stopped just in time for the wind to quit blowing, and it caught me leaning with my feet still attached to the pedal. In my mind, I think I looked like Artie Johnson on his tricycle on the old *Laugh-In* television show. After picking myself up and dusting off, the following conversation ensued.

Chad: Are you okay?

Me: Yes, I think so.

Chad: Are you sure?

Me: Except for my pride, I'm fine.

Chad: Good. That means I can laugh. That was the funniest thing I've ever seen.

One Sunday after church, Chad and I took off for a ride up to the north part of McKinney. We had reached Highway 75 and were crossing over to the northbound frontage road. Chad suggested we turn left and head north on the frontage road. I followed his left turn, and we headed downhill. This section of frontage road goes downhill and then does a U-turn under 75 and then heads uphill on the southbound side. I realized too late where we were and that I'd have to climb back up the other side. I hate climbing.

Me: Hey, if we go down this side, don't we have to go up the other side?

Chad: Yes.

Me: You jerk!

Laughing, Chad rides away.

———

After work, whenever possible, I like to take a quick ten- to fifteen-mile ride to relax. One particular evening both boys decided to accompany me. As usual in Texas during the summer, the wind was blowing hard out of the south. We made a turn, and the wind hit us in the face. We hadn't gone very far when I realized that neither of the boys was at my side. I took a quick look over my shoulder. They were riding single file behind me.

Me: Hey, what are you guys doing?

Them: Drafting.

Me: Why?

Them: You make a good wind break.

Me: Jerks.

Them: (laughing)

———

Well, there you have it—a few of my favorite memories. When I ride with the boys, I'm never quite sure where we will go or how we'll get there, but I know it will be fun and that I'll cherish the time. I'm blessed and proud to call them my sons. I don't know what the next months or years hold for me, but I know that my wingmen will be there to lift my spirits.

Love you guys.

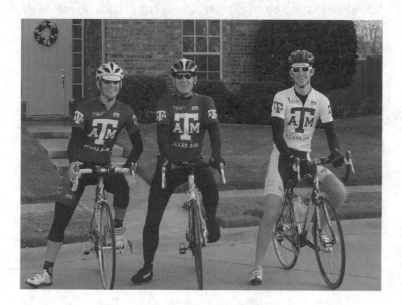

THE SYCAMORE TREE

August 10, 2010

I came down with bronchitis over the weekend and have been coughing and not sleeping at night. Both nights, a particular event that occurred just before my symptoms began to appear has been playing over and over in my mind.

Do you ever have songs just pop into your mind from nowhere? We laugh about it around the house when it happens. DeLayne seems to have old classic hymns running through her head, and I have old vacation Bible school kid songs playing in mine. That should probably tell you something about the difference between DeLayne's musical talents and my own.

One morning as I was backing out of the driveway, the kid song about Zacchaeus popped into my head. The story of Zacchaeus is detailed in Luke 19. Some of you may have learned this song and might be humming along now. It's probably been forty years since I sang that song, but there were those lyrics just like it was yesterday.

Why was this song suddenly stuck in my mind? I could have just passed it off, but it kept happening day after day for several days. Then one morning, I heard the radio announcer say, "Remember, today you may be the only Jesus someone sees." Just like that, the puzzle pieces fell into place and led me to ask myself a rather haunting question. *If my life were a sycamore tree, would someone crossing my path be able to climb it and see Jesus?* Sadly, the answer to that question is no. There have been times in my life that if people were to climb that tree, they wouldn't catch a glimpse of Jesus. Thankfully, and praise God, I'm forgiven!

Since that morning, I've had a new morning prayer. Each morning, I ask God to grant me the grace that whoever may cross my path that day would see Jesus in my words, actions, and deeds. I've been finding it easier to be courteous and forgiving to people as I go through the day. I thought I'd found the deep meaning in this song.

Then came the diagnoses of cancer. Now there's a new branch in my sycamore tree. I realize now there will be multiple people coming into my life on a daily basis—doctors, nurses, lab techs, and other cancer patients. So now I have another prayer. I pray for God to heal me and for people to be able to see Jesus in me during the process.

EYE OF THE STORM

August 19, 2010

We've just completed our first day at MD Anderson Cancer Center (MDA). DeLayne asked me after we got back to the hotel if I ever felt anxious today.

"No, I never really did."

Part of that may have been due to having DeLayne's brother and sister-in-law here in Houston to show us the ropes. It helps when you've had people who have gone before you help lead you into the battle.

Another part of it is this constant feeling I have that God has been laying the foundation for the events to come for many, many years. Take, for instance, DeLayne getting the urge to reconnect with friends from twenty years ago. Turns out that some of them have fought the cancer battle and now call or email their prayers and encouragement. Or the young lady I met in Bangkok almost twelve years ago who moved to the United States. This young lady walked into my office two days after the diagnosis and asked if she could pray for me. These are just two of the instances that confirm to me that God has a plan and will give me the peace and grace to fight this battle. I've tried to describe to friends the sense of calm that both DeLayne and I feel, but the only way I can think of is to say we're living in the eye of the storm. Where we are right now is calm.

There's a great story in the Bible about Peter, my favorite disciple. The disciples have all gotten into a boat to sail to the other side of the sea. Jesus has stayed behind for the evening.

In the middle of the night, the disciples see a figure walking on the water. At first, they believe it to be a spirit but then realize it's Jesus. Peter calls out to Him and tells Jesus that if it's really Him to say so, and he will come out to Him. The next thing Peter knows, he's out of the boat and walking on the water. Everything is fine until Peter takes his eyes off Jesus. Peter notices the wind and the clouds and starts to sink. He calls out to Jesus, and Jesus takes his hand and pulls Peter back to the surface.

This story has really struck home with me the last few weeks. As long as I keep my focus on Jesus daily, I don't see the storm around me, and I sense the calmness of His love for me. But if I try to look too far ahead, all I see are the rolling, boiling storm clouds, and I feel scared with the uncertainty of it all.

If doubt is going to find its way in, it will come in the night. That's when everyone is in bed, the house is quiet, and I'm alone with my thoughts. My almost nightly prayer is for Jesus to hold me close when I'm scared and be my Prince of Peace.

PEPPER

August 26, 2010

There's no sense pretending that yesterday wasn't the lowest point of this battle so far. It was then that we found out I have stage IV lung cancer. That pretty much took the wind right out of my sails. I spent last evening calling family and letting them know what we had learned and that I was scheduled for yet another round of biopsies this week. I went to bed praying for just a little good news.

This morning brought a new day with new challenges. DeLayne wanted to attend a class at MD Anderson, and she left me alone in the hotel. Honestly, at that point, I just wanted to curl up on the couch and cry, but something made me get up and get out my camera and start yet another project I've been planning. While preparing my camera, I kept asking God for something—anything—that would make me chuckle.

Across the street from our hotel is a small park with fountains. I made my way over there to see if there was anything to photograph. I had taken just a couple of photos when I noticed a guy walking his dog by one of the fountains. We said good morning to each other as we passed. When I got to the end of the fountain, I turned around and saw his dog running into the water. This fountain has spouts that shoot the water straight up. I watched as this dog started trying to catch the water. The next thing I knew, I was laughing at what I was watching as the dog ran from spout to spout. I thought I needed some photos of this and went back to ask the owner if it would be okay to photograph his dog. He gave permission and introduced me to Pepper.

Pepper is a rescue dog and is, oddly, afraid of water. I guess that includes lakes and swimming pools, because with fountains, she was having a lot of fun and kept going back for more. Pepper may have been a rescue dog, but today she was a four-legged angel. I spent the next several minutes photographing and watching Pepper.

After they left, I took a few more pictures around the park before getting a call that I had an appointment to get back in the battle—but now I had a much better attitude.

I realized that today I had asked God for a chuckle, and He gave me Pepper.

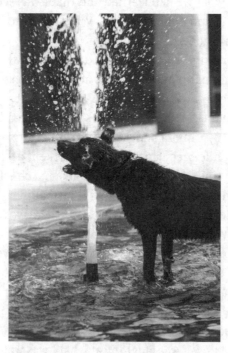

CHANGES

September 19, 2010

I think it's part of human nature to resist changes to the way we do things, or maybe I should say it's part of my nature to resist. Starting from the day I was diagnosed with cancer, I've been determined to not allow cancer to change or significantly alter my life. I wanted life to continue on as normal, whatever *normal* could possibly mean. As hard as I was trying, I began to suspect that cancer was changing my normal when I walked into church last Sunday morning. The side effects from the Tarceva chemotherapy treatment had started to appear. I found myself deciding where to sit so I could leave, if necessary, without disrupting the service for those around me. My suspicions were confirmed Thursday morning when I entered the MDA radiation clinic and saw emblazoned on a waiting room television, "Cancer changes everything." Since then, I've been reflecting over the past months to see how else cancer has changed my life.

At first glance, there have been changes that appear positive but are actually negative. For some time now, I've been trying to lose some weight. Ordinarily, I'd feel good about losing twenty pounds and an inch off my waist. I know a lot of people who have paid a lot of money for those kinds of results, but this is not a weight-loss plan I'd wish on anyone. Eating all the time and not gaining weight is good for a teenager, but I have to eat every few hours to keep from losing more weight. Sometimes, I actually get tired of eating.

Then there are changes that appear to be negative but are actually proving to have positive results. The lung tumor has caused part of my lung to collapse. This makes it difficult to speak sometimes. Singing is all but out of the question. Not being able to sing may be a positive for those around me, but I'm finding it also has a positive effect on me. Since I can't sing, I'm now more closely reading the words to the hymns, and I'm realizing what a wonderful gift the old hymns are to the church. Don't tell your music ministers I said this, but try this sometime: Stop singing and read the words. Let them soak in.

Finally, there are changes that can only be seen as positive. Sunrises and sunsets no longer just mark the beginning and ending of each day. They are times to be thankful for another day and celebrate the glory of God's creation. I know that my prayers and talks with God are a bit more direct and urgent. My quiet times and Bible study times are deeper now. I love Jesus and appreciate what He has done for me more than ever. I love and value my sons more now than the day they were born. I love my wife more each day and 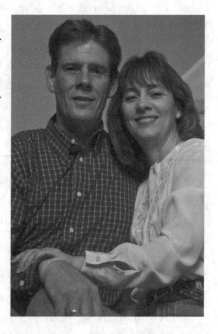 thank God every day that she's here for me to lean on. I simply can't imagine going through this without her by my side.

FINDING THE RIGHT GEAR

October 3, 2010

Whenever I get to ride my bicycle, I notice there are times the pedaling seems effortless. There's a natural rhythm to my legs and breathing. That's when I know I've found the right gear. A lot of life is the same way. We find ourselves in a rhythm, and we just roll through the day feeling good about our lives. Then something comes along and knocks us out of our natural rhythm. We find ourselves desperately looking for any way to find it again. On a bike, that's when I realize I'm riding uphill in way too big of a gear.

For me, fighting cancer is very similar. I begin to feel better when I can find the rhythm between taking the medicine, eating, sleeping, and other daily activities. My biggest problem up until now has been finding that rhythm and staying in it. Every time I think I'm about to find the right gear, something else comes along and knocks me out of my rhythm. Pneumonia has been the culprit for the last two weeks. Then, just when I think I have the pneumonia under control, the side effects from some of the medicines kick in, and I have to start all over again.

Last Tuesday was a day that I had to start over again. Monday had gone well, and I was beginning to feel like I was getting there. Then Monday evening, I noticed a strange taste to my food. Then just like that, everything started tasting bad. Tuesday morning, I had to force down my breakfast, and I could feel my energy level begin to drop from the lack of food.

As I got in my truck and headed to work, I began to ask myself if this was ever going to end. It was during this drive I realized I was pedaling uphill in way too big a gear. I was one stop light away from turning around, going back home to bed, and pulling the covers over my head. As if on cue, a song by Casting Crowns came on the radio that fit me perfectly: "Praise You in This Storm." I was reminded Who is large and in charge.

God used this song to provide the kick in the pants I needed and remind me that no matter the circumstances, I'm to look to Him for help and praise Him. I won't lie to you and tell you that right now I'm able to praise God for cancer, but slowly, He's teaching me to give Him praise in the midst of this storm.

Sometimes the problem isn't the gear you're in—it's who's pedaling the bike.

BLESSED ASSURANCE

October 10, 2010

Well, here I sit. In slightly less than forty-eight hours, I'll again be injected with a radioactive glucose solution and placed in a machine to be scanned from the tip of my nose to my belly button. The results of the scan will show if the lung cancer has continued to advance or if we have struck a blow against this beast in my chest. As I think about this, I can't help but think that I should feel more anxious about this next week. But strangely, I don't. I've shared before how I was told that the battle would be long and hard but that I would be healed. Even since that time, God has continued to give me assurances that eventually I will be healed. I pray daily that He would let me in on the timeline and plan, but He has chosen not to do that. Until such time He chooses to give me more details, I'll have to live with the assurances He's given me.

One morning after beginning the Tarceva cancer treatment, I could feel fatigue beginning to set in. I had finished my morning devotional reading and asked God to give me a little extra for the day. The Bible that I use is the *Life Application Study Bible*. At the beginning of each book, there's an introduction and blueprint for that book. After asking God for the little extra, I randomly opened my Bible. I looked down to see that my Bible had opened to the introduction to Matthew. I thought I must have missed by a page or two and flipped back and forth. Not seeing anything else, I had decided to just close my Bible and get on with my day.

That's when I heard this slightly exasperated voice in my head say, *Just read the introduction.* As I read, I remember thinking to myself, *What does this have to do with fighting cancer?* As soon as I reached the final paragraph, my eyes began to tear.

The words were:

As you read this Gospel, listen to Matthew's clear message: Jesus is the Christ, the King of kings and Lord of lords. Celebrate his victory over evil and death, and make Jesus the Lord of your life.[1]

Jesus has already fought this battle for me. I look forward to the day we can rejoice in His victory.

After coming home from the hospital from a bout with pneumonia, I was unable to get comfortable in bed. Instead of lying there thinking whatever random thoughts popped into my head, I decided to get up. After reading a little from another book, I felt I should read my Bible. I said a prayer along the lines of, "God, I'm not feeling too well tonight. Please show me something that there are better days ahead." I opened my Bible and there, before my eyes, was this verse.

"But for you who fear My name, the sun of righteousness will rise with healing in its wings; and you will go forth and skip about like calves from the stall."

—MALACHI 4:2

That, my friends, brings a whole new meaning to sunrise.

The Bible talks about angels and how we are each given one. I actually saw mine. I was going through diagnostic testing in Houston. Early one morning, I was asleep in the hotel room. I

---

[1] *Life Application Study Bible, NASB* (Grand Rapids, MI: Zondervan, 2000), 1578.

was dreaming I was in the same hotel room and facing the door to the bedroom. Suddenly, I realized there was a man standing in the doorway. I remember thinking, *Why is that man in the doorway?* He was dressed in either a robe or gown that was tied at the waist. Slowly, he walked across the room to my side of the bed. As I looked at him, he bent over and laid his hand on my chest. The sensation of being touched was so real it startled me awake. I've thought about this for several weeks, trying to figure out what it all meant. I've finally concluded this was my guardian angel simply telling me he's in this battle with me and watching over me.

As I head into this next week, I'm leaning on these blessed assurances to determine what direction we go next.

FRIENDS

October 13, 2010

Do you ever stop and think about the people you call friends? I'm not sure I've ever really given it much thought. I know there are some people I hold a little closer than others. With the way things are today, people just come and go through our lives. We move on and make new friends. Some friends we stay in touch with because our lives are intertwined. Others just stay on our Christmas card list.

One thing I'm learning is that DeLayne and I have great friends. We have friends that come mow our yard and take care of our house while we're gone. Friends have brought us snacks or meals to show us they care. Some of our friends have a knack for showing up when they know we need a laugh or a hug. Others seem to know when we can use a phone call to check up on us or an email to encourage us.

I've wondered how these friends know what we need when we need it. My only explanation is God prompts them. During my last quiet time, I read a Bible verse that perfectly describes this kind of friendship. In Philippians, there are some great verses for cancer patients:

I have learned to be content in whatever circumstances I am. . . . I can do all things through Him who strengthens me.
—PHILIPPIANS 4:11, 13

But in verse 14, Paul describes the kind of friends that DeLayne and I have:

Nevertheless, you have done well to share with me in my affliction.

Notice that he says, "In my affliction." These are the friends that are in the battle with you. These are the kind of friends that we are blessed to have surrounding us now.

If there was one piece of advice I could give young people, it would be this: Build your life with and surround yourselves with the kind of friends that will share in your afflictions. They will make a difference in your life.

HOPE: PART 1

October 20, 2010

I apologize if you've been checking to see anything new and just find the same old news. After learning that the Tarceva didn't work, I needed a break. I had grown wary of building my hopes up just to see them dashed on the cold, hard rocks of reality. Each time, I would rebuild just to find there were pieces missing. I awoke one morning with the idea in my head that if I was looking for hope, I should start with the Bible. I decided to look up each verse with the word "hope," write it in my notebook, and then write my feelings and thoughts about each verse. In my Bible version, there are thirty-one verses in twenty-one different books of the Bible. Here are some of those verses with what I wrote.

"Where now is my hope? And who regards my hope?"
—JOB 17:15

I know just how Job feels. I feel like all of the hope I had when this started is being slowly drained away from me. I need something to plug the hole.

For the needy will not always be forgotten, nor the hope of the afflicted perish forever.
—PSALM 9:18

At this point, I'd consider myself one of the needy. I need some good news; healing would be great. I feel like I've been forgotten. Is God hearing me? I would also say that I'm afflicted. My hope will not perish forever. I just pray that God sends a lifeline soon.

"And now, Lord, for what do I wait? My hope is in You."
—Psalm 39:7

The bottom line is, I'm losing faith in the doctors and medicine. Why am I the guy that things don't work for? I have to put my hope in the Lord to provide the healing.

For You are my hope; O Lord God, You are my confidence from my youth.
—Psalm 71:5

When I look back through my life, it's easy to see where God worked on my behalf. Is He working today? Is He trying to bring me to the point where I recognize He is all the hope I have?

Discipline your son while there is hope, and do not desire his death.
—Proverbs 19:18

Is God disciplining me? Part of the word "discipline" is "disciple." In all of this frustration and disappointment, is God trying to teach me something? I must be a slow learner. I wish He would hurry and finish the lesson, or, at least, let me peek at the lesson plan.

He doesn't desire my death. God's desire is for me to be completely healed. I guess the healing will come after the lesson is complete.

O Lord, the hope of Israel, all who forsake You will be put to shame. Because they have forsaken the fountain of living water, even the Lord.
—Jeremiah 17:13

Could it be there is someone witnessing my struggle who has turned away from the Lord? Will He eventually use my healing to draw them back? I need to find this person and give them a hug.

The Lord is the fountain of living water. I need a long, cool drink!

———

Well, there are the first few verses. I'll admit to having more questions than answers. I have faith that God will answer them in His timing as we continue our journey down this road called cancer.

HOPE: PART 2

October 22, 2010 (Morning)
Before Being Sent to the Emergency Room

Then He said to me, "Son of man, these bones are the whole house of Israel; behold, they say, 'Our bones are dried up and our hope has perished. We are completely cut off.'"

—EZEKIEL 37:11

I'm not feeling well again. My temperature is up, and my legs hurt. The pneumonia is back, I think. Every time this happens, I feel more of my hope perish. Why do I have to have lung cancer *and* pneumonia? God, one of them would be enough! Please fix one or the other soon. I'm tired of being miserable.

But perceiving that one group were Sadducees and the other Pharisees, Paul began crying out in the Council, "Brethren, I am a Pharisee, a son of Pharisees; I am on trial for the hope and resurrection of the dead!"

—ACTS 23:6

Hope of the dead, Jesus is our hope. But I feel that with each day that passes, this cancer is sucking the life out of me. Please God, let us get the upper hand on it soon.

And hope does not disappoint, because the love of God has been poured out within our hearts through the Holy Spirit who was given to us.

—ROMANS 5:5

This is the last verse in a series. Verses 3–4 talk about being exulted in our tribulation because they will bring about perseverance, and perseverance brings hope. With each tribulation I persevere (pneumonia, chemo, IV sticks, and PICC lines), my hope will increase. Right now, it doesn't feel that way. Every high seems lower and every low seems lower. Please God, have the Holy Spirit give me more hope.

Rejoicing in hope, persevering in tribulation, devoted to prayer.

—ROMANS 12:12

When my hope is drained, I don't feel like rejoicing. Maybe I have it backward. Maybe if I start rejoicing, my hope will be restored. I must praise Him in the storm.

HOPE: PART 3

October 22, 2010 (Evening)
In the Hospital

Now may the God of hope fill you with all joy and peace in believing, so that you will abound in hope by the power of the Holy Spirit.

—ROMANS 15:13

God is the God of hope! He will fill me with joy and peace as I continue to believe. My hope is that God will heal me. I will only abide in hope by the power of the Holy Spirit and none other.

Or is He speaking altogether for our sake? Yes, for our sake it was written, because the plowman ought to plow in hope, and the thresher to thresh in hope of sharing the crops.

—1 CORINTHIANS 9:10

Is God wanting to use me as a plowman? Am I plowing fields now with hope of reaching people for Him? Will all of this end in the sharing of the crop that is Jesus?

But now faith, hope, love, abide these three; but the greatest of these is love.

—1 CORINTHIANS 13:13

I have faith and hope that I will be healed. I know Jesus loves me. I know lots of other people love me and are praying for me daily. I need to keep the faith, rebuild my hope, and surround myself with people who love me.

For we through the Spirit, by faith, are waiting for the hope of righteousness.

—GALATIANS 5:5

I must keep my faith in Jesus to see me through the days and weeks ahead and hope for the righteousness that awaits on the other side.

I pray that the eyes of your heart may be enlightened, so that you will know what is the hope of His calling, what are the riches of the glory of His inheritance in the saints.

—EPHESIANS 1:18

God, open my heart so I may see hope in what You are calling me into. I want to share in the glory of Your inheritance.

If indeed you continue in the faith firmly established and steadfast, and not moved away from the hope of the gospel that you have heard, which was proclaimed in all creation under heaven, and of which I, Paul, was made a minister.

—COLOSSIANS 1:23

Jesus is the hope of the gospel. No matter what is coming my way, I'll remain steadfast in that belief.

HOPE: PART 4

October 23, 2010

To whom God willed to make known what is the riches of the glory of this mystery among the Gentiles, which is Christ in you, the hope of glory.

—COLOSSIANS 1:27

Christ living in me may be a mystery to the rest of the world, but I know He is here. He is my hope and glory.

But since we are of the day, let us be sober, having put on the breastplate of faith and love, and as a helmet, the hope of salvation.

—1 THESSALONIANS 5:8

It's interesting that the two battle garments in this verse cover the head and chest. The two places that cancer has attacked my body are covered by faith and the hope of salvation—Jesus.

So that being justified by His grace we would be made heirs according to the hope of eternal life.

—TITUS 3:7

I have been justified by God's grace and Jesus' death on the cross. I now have the hope of eternal life. If I don't beat cancer here, I'll beat it there.

Blessed be the God and Father of our Lord Jesus Christ, who according to His great mercy has caused us to be born again to a living hope through the resurrection of Jesus Christ from the dead.

—1 PETER 1:3

God has great mercy for his children, and I now have a living hope that can't be taken away. Even cancer will not take that hope away.

But sanctify Christ as Lord in your hearts, always being ready to make a defense to everyone who asks you to give an account for the hope that is in you, yet with gentleness and reverence.

—1 PETER 3:15

My hope is Jesus. I need to be prepared to share that hope with others. Maybe God will use this cancer and my blog to let others know of my hope in Jesus.

HOPE: PART 5

October 24, 2010

Though He slay me, I will hope in Him. Nevertheless I will argue my ways before Him.

—JOB 13:15

Job is saying that no matter what, his hope is in God. He is still going to make his case to God. I feel the same way. I plead my case to God daily. I want things to be the way they were, but that will never happen.

For I hope in You, O LORD; You will answer, O Lord my God.

—PSALM 38:15

I hope in the Lord, also. I know He's answering prayers daily for me. The big one remains unanswered. I'm praying I will be healed of the pneumonia just so I can breathe easier and start chemo.

All of us growl like bears, and moan sadly like doves; We hope for justice, but there is none, for salvation, but it is far from us.

—ISAIAH 59:11

I hope and pray for justice. I don't believe it is just for me to have cancer. I feel there's no justice every time I cough. Unlike Isaiah, though, I feel my salvation is near.

Give glory to the LORD your God, before He brings darkness and before your feet stumble on the dusky mountains, and while you are hoping for light He makes it into deep darkness, and turns it into gloom.

—JEREMIAH 13:16

Can it really get darker and gloomier? It couldn't get any lower than lunch today in the hospital when Chad and Shane had to help feed me. It's not supposed to be like this so early in their lives. I keep hoping for light, but it keeps getting darker.

"AND IN HIS NAME THE GENTILES WILL HOPE."

—MATTHEW 12:21

My hope is in the name of Jesus. I know that He's working. The brain tumor has been successfully treated. Can we please take care of the pneumonia and start treating the lung cancer?

[Love] bears all things, believes all things, hopes all things, endures all things.

—1 CORINTHIANS 13:7

This verse is speaking of love. Boy, is it true. DeLayne has to bear a lot from me. Like me, she's hoping for healing. Only God knows what our love will have to endure before this is over.

HOPE: PART 6

October 25, 2010

We who were the first to hope in Christ would be to the praise of His glory.

—EPHESIANS 1:12

Again, my hope is in Christ. Someday, I'll give praise in His glory. I pray that His glory is shown here on earth by my complete healing.

But I hope in the Lord Jesus to send Timothy to you shortly, so that I also may be encouraged when I learn of your condition.

—PHILIPPIANS 2:19

Is there a Timothy for me? I need to hear some encouraging news. Or, does God plan to use me as someone's Timothy to encourage them? I don't know the answer. God hasn't made His plan evident to me. I wish He would!

Now faith is the assurance of things hoped for, the conviction of things not seen.

—HEBREWS 11:1

I'm hoping and praying I will be healed. My faith in Jesus assures me that someday it will happen, even though right now, I can't see that day.

Though I have many things to write to you, I do not want to do so with paper and ink; but I hope to come to you and speak face to face, so that your joy may be made full.

—2 JOHN 12

There is someone in my future that I'll have to speak with face-to-face for them to believe that I'm completely healed. At that time, their joy will be made full. Will this person then find a new or renewed love of Christ?

STINKIN' THINKIN'

November 6, 2010

Looking back through my notes on the verses about hope, I noticed some items that can only be described as stinkin' thinkin'. I had grown frustrated and was emotionally down. I had climbed up on my pity pot and gotten comfortable. Satan used this opportunity to pounce like the lion he is and plant ideas about God that just aren't true.

The idea that I've had recently that has unsettled me the most is the thought that God has chosen not to heal my cancer or relieve any of the symptoms because there's a lesson He wants me to learn. *What?* The only thing I can think of to compare this line of thinking to is that of a father and son. The father has told his son not to do something but, as boys are inclined to do, he does it anyway. The result is that he breaks his arm. To teach his son a lesson on obedience, the father decides not to take his son to the doctor for two days. We all recognize immediately this father is abusive. Yet, we have no problem assigning those same attributes to God.

How many times have we thought God has allowed bad circumstances to come into our lives to teach us a lesson? I'm not talking about suffering the consequences of our choices but about things we have no control over, like cancer. I'm convinced God desires the best for me and for me to be completely healed and whole again. In the Bible, Jesus even says, "Or what man is there among you who, when his son asks for a loaf, will give him a stone? Or if he asks for a fish, he will not give him a snake, will he?" (Matthew 7:9–10).

I'm going to have to bind Satan daily to keep this kind of stinkin' thinkin' in check.

Some of you may be thinking to yourselves that I'm being a little tough on myself. I've been convicted that I simply can't allow this kind of thinking to enter my mind and comments. During my study of the verses about hope, there were several verses that spoke of people who had lost their hope in Jesus or wandered away from God. Jesus wants His relationship with these people restored. From the reading of these verses, I'm burdened with the thought that they are watching me and probably reading what I write here. I have to be mindful of that and be sure that nothing I say, do, or write validates their belief that God doesn't love them or care for them.

Another thing I've learned the past few weeks is that cancer isn't just a physical battle. It's a mental and spiritual battle as well. I will daily have to put on armor to fight the battle with cancer. God may use the doctors, nurses, medicines, and procedures as tools that lead to healing, but in the end, God will use faith, love, and hope to provide complete healing.

God isn't using cancer to teach me a lesson, but, eventually, He will use my healing to teach Satan a lesson.

I'LL TELL YOU A SECRET

November 11, 2010

Last Sunday some good friends, David and Cindy, brought us dinner. We had a few minutes to visit and reminisce about summers spent together at baseball fields. Cindy then complimented me on this blog and my writing. I had to confess my secret to her then, and I'll confess to you now, that I almost failed freshman composition in college. The teacher didn't like anything I wrote, sent me to writer's lab, and encouraged me to drop the class. I stuck it out because I just couldn't see going through the pain and suffering again. Honestly, most of my life I haven't had the talent and rarely the desire to write much more than "Happy Birthday" in a card.

Why is it important for you to know this? Because I want you to know that I can't take credit for this blog. I can't explain how the day after I was diagnosed with lung cancer, the desire hit me to start writing. This has to be a God thing. I asked God for some good to come out of this cancer. Suddenly, I have this platform. Some of the topics I write about come to me in the middle of the night. Others come while I'm lying on a table being treated or tested. Some topics are almost completely written as soon as the idea comes. Others take a few days to think through. I'm never quite sure where a blog will go sometimes but trust God will give me the words I need. Each time I post, I pray God will use the blog to touch someone in a special way. I enjoy when people leave comments or send me emails, because that means prayers are being answered.

I've always felt God has a plan in all of this. The fact that I'm writing this blog convinces me of this. I'm not sure where the plan will lead but know God will use this for good. Although I don't know for how long God will give me this platform, I'll continue to use it for as long as He allows me to do so. I never thought His plan would include writing a blog.

I'm reminded to always be open to where God wants to lead.

AREA FIFTY-ONE

November 17, 2010

Well, here it is. Today is my fifty-first birthday. I'm officially now over the hill. I'm praying for a long, smooth descent. I've spent the last few days thinking about and comparing what was supposed to be against what has become and shedding a few tears. My fifty-first birthday wasn't supposed to be about radiation treatments, chemotherapy, MRIs, and CT scans, but it is. DeLayne asked me what I wanted for my birthday. All I could think of was for this to be gone.

Fifty-one years have gone by faster than I thought they could. How many things have I postponed, thinking that I would do them later? Now I wonder, *Will "later" ever come?* Since the reality of today no longer matches the dreams of yesterday, and I don't know what tomorrow holds, I will spend time reflecting and counting my blessings.

One thing I can't deny is how richly blessed my life has been. To have been born in this country to Christian parents who taught us the difference between needs and wants is more than what most of the world has been blessed with. We were never a wealthy family, but we never went hungry. There was always a roof over our heads and clothes on our back. Being raised with five siblings may not have always been seen as a blessing growing up, but now I'm thankful for all of them. As my mother told my brother and me after our dad's first heart attack, "You kids are all different and don't always get along, but when someone in this family needs help, you're there for each other." Mom and Dad are both gone now and enjoying their rewards, but the legacy of their children remains. I'm blessed to call them my family.

I've been blessed to work for the same company twenty-five years now. Looking back through those years, I can see how God always had a hand on my career. The right opportunities always appeared at the right times. My job has allowed me to go places and see things that others just dream about. There were times I had to make a choice between seeking advancement and family, but I don't recall ever making the wrong choice. My job has allowed us to enjoy family vacations that will forever be locked in our memories. We are able to send both boys to college and have enjoyed watching them grow and mature while there. We can look forward with great expectations as to what God has planned for their lives.

Last, but not least, I've been blessed with a wife like none other and two great sons. DeLayne and I have been married for twenty-six years now. She's become my rock to lean on. After all these years, we think so much alike, it can be scary at times. Now we've learned that the dinner dishes can wait. Just sitting on the couch holding each other is more important. Chad and Shane have both grown up to be fine young men. Both of them have great instincts about when I could use a little tweak or when to call just to cheer me up. They will someday change the world because they won't accept it the way it is. I look forward to watching them both race in France someday.

I keep telling DeLayne, "I haven't had my midlife crisis yet; I should be good for at least fifty-one more years."

Yes, I've been truly been blessed during my lifetime. This blog today is probably more for me than for you. I need to be reminded from time to time that God has been so good to me and will continue to be so. Although I'm fifty-one, I'll spend my day much like a little child curled up in his grandfather's lap, held securely in his arms. I will be secure in the loving arms and lap of God, knowing that He knit me together in my mother's womb. Only He knows the number of my days and the plans He has to prosper me, to further bless me, and to heal me.

REAR-VIEW MIRRORS

November 21, 2010

We all know what rear-view mirrors are. They are those annoying things attached to our cars that show us where we've been. We're in too big a hurry charging ahead with places to go and people to see to worry about what we've left behind. We only check the rear-view mirrors to see if those flashing lights behind are for us. I've recognized over the past few months that God has blessed each of us with a rear-view mirror in our minds. They call it "memory." Unfortunately, we don't use this one very often, either. Over these past few weeks, I've had ample opportunities to check my rear-view mirror while lying on the radiation treatment table.

On Friday morning, October 22, after receiving the news that the MRI showed good results concerning the brain tumor, I was immediately sent to the MDA emergency room with a high fever. I was officially admitted to the hospital later that night and wasn't a happy camper. I was receiving intravenous (IV) antibiotics every few hours. With each IV change came the question, *Why is this happening again?* I was still confident that God had a plan, but I was beginning to lose confidence in the plan. My faith was being stretched to new lengths.

There were two significant things that happened that weekend. First, the oncologist on call correctly diagnosed what was happening to me and recommended a complete change in my treatment plan to include radiation treatments that started two days later. Second, this doctor was informed about a new lung cancer mutation that was being found in never-smokers who had tested negative for the other two known mutations. The new genetic mutation, named EML4-ALK ("ALK" for short), is known to exist in only 3 to 7 percent of all lung cancer patients. The doctor was taking the proverbial shot in the dark, but he was recommending that my biopsies be sent for analysis. Test results would take six to eight weeks.

On November 16, I completed the recommended radiation treatments. On November 17, my birthday, God gave me a present of a lifetime. In less than four weeks, the mutation test results came back. I was positive for the ALK gene mutation. The enemy in my chest now has a name. We are no longer fighting the unknown. The battle and journey are far from over, but now we have a map.

Looking in my rear-view mirror, I can see that God knew well in advance the doctor who would be on duty, his capabilities, and his knowledge. Too often I forget my simple prayer that God put the right people in the right place at the right time. Once again, He has been faithful to supply that person.

Thinking about the rear-view mirror in my truck, I remember it has a compass in it. Sometimes you have to look backward to build your faith that God knows the direction going forward.

IT'S A WONDERFUL LIFE

November 28, 2010

Every year between Thanksgiving and Christmas, there are three movies I have to watch: *White Christmas, Miracle on 34th Street*, and *It's a Wonderful Life*. Of the three, *It's a Wonderful Life* is my favorite. I'm not sure why. I guess the movie just speaks to me. It doesn't matter how many times I watch this movie, I still tear up at the end when all of George's friends come to help him out. The other thing could be because this movie asks the question we've all asked from time to time, *Would it matter to anyone if I weren't here?*

If you haven't seen the movie, George is the main character. He's gone through life giving up his hopes and dreams in order to help others. He finds himself in a particularly difficult financial situation. At the end of his rope, he says, "Maybe it would have been better if I had never been born." Clarence, his angel, decides to teach him a lesson and show him what life would have been like for all his friends had he not been born. George finally realizes the error of his thinking and decides to live on. Back in his life, all of George's friends come to help him, and he gets out of his financial difficulties. Most importantly, George realizes he's made a difference in the world.

The first ten or fifteen times I watched this movie, my question was the same as George's: *Would anyone notice if I weren't here?* The last few times I've watched the movie though, I've found myself asking a different question. Now I ask, *Have I made a difference to anyone?* When I ask this question, my focus begins to change. I find that when I ask this question, my pockets always have extra money when I walk by the red kettle for donations. It becomes a little easier to feel sorry for the mother whose child wants everything in the store. When I leave the stores, I'm reminded to smile and say, "Have a merry Christmas" to the clerks—even if they aren't allowed to say it back.

This year between Thanksgiving and Christmas, let's all try to make a difference.

In closing, let me say that there are a lot of people who, if you weren't here, the Haga family would miss. Thanks for being there.

MY PSALM

December 13, 2010

I've been reading a book where the author comments about the importance of personalizing Scripture. After having delayed chemotherapy for the second time, I prayed that God would prepare me for yet a third time. I felt led to begin reading ten psalms each morning and underlining parts that touched me. I then read back the underlined portions to God as my morning prayer. I'm surprised each morning at the prayer that emerges from the verses. I've yet to make it through a single prayer without weeping.

There are other psalms where I'll replace a few words. These are becoming the psalms that God is using to prepare me for my upcoming treatments. The psalms of David are the ones that seem to translate the easiest. David was tormented by his enemies and his own sins, and he always poured his heart out to God. One morning, Psalm 27:1 was in my reading. As I read the first verse, a few new words popped into my head. My new psalm reads like this: "The LORD is my light and my salvation; *What* shall I fear? The LORD is the defense of my life; *What treatment* shall I dread?"

So with these words on my lips and in my heart, God is preparing me for the next leg in this journey to defeat cancer. Only He knows what lies ahead on this path. I'm assured He has gone before me and is my light and defender.

THE PROCESS

January 8, 2011

During the diagnosis phase, I asked my pulmonologist some questions concerning what may lay ahead. He answered me with, "You have to understand that you've started a process. There are many steps that will have to be taken in a particular order, and each will take time." Of course, he was speaking from the medical perspective. Over the last few months, I've started to learn this is also true from a spiritual perspective as well.

While I was recovering from the radiation treatments and preparing to begin chemotherapy, I completed my study of the book of Psalms. During this time, I became even more convinced I'll be healed from cancer. This conviction led me to ask the following question of God: *If You're going to heal me, why put me through radiation, chemo, and all of these tests and treatments? Why not just heal me now?*

Then one morning when I woke up, the first thing to come to mind was Lazarus. That thought seemed out of place with what I'd been reading, so I ignored it and pushed it out of my mind. I'll admit I'm not the sharpest tack in the box sometimes, but when it happened two more mornings, I finally took the hint and opened my Bible to the story of Lazarus in John 11 and 12.

The first thing I noticed is that Jesus knew the sickness wouldn't end in death but for the glory of God, and so the

Son of God would be glorified. Also, even though Jesus loved Lazarus, He waited to go to him.

I, too, will wait so the Son of God will be glorified in my healing. I'll admit I don't like waiting. I want this process to move faster than it is, but at each phase of my treatment, we learn something new that we wouldn't have learned if we were moving faster.

The second thing I noticed is Lazarus' sisters stated a variation of my question to Jesus. "If you had come sooner, you could have healed him." Jesus tries to explain to them about the resurrection and life. When they and the crowds with them continue to weep, He sees their doubt and is deeply troubled.

It strikes me that my question shows I also have some doubt about God's plan and the process He's putting me through. Sometimes doubt enters my thoughts, but I still maintain the faith in my heart. The one thing I don't want to do is grieve Jesus with my doubt.

The final thing I noticed is that the chief priest started making plans to kill Lazarus. Why? Because he had become a witness for Jesus. Large crowds were gathering to see him. This part makes me smile a little. I like to imagine Lazarus being at dinner or out on the street, and a large crowd gathers to look at him. Finally, someone musters the courage to ask him, "Hey, aren't you the Lazarus that died?" And he answers, "Yes, I am, and let me tell you what Jesus did for me."

This makes me look forward to the day that someone comes up to me and says, "Hey, aren't you the Chris Haga who had lung cancer?" And I can answer, "Yes, I am, and let me tell you what Jesus did for me."

Most of all, through all of this, I'm learning that God has a plan for the rest of my life. He only reveals to me what I need to know for each day. It's become evident to me that part of the plan includes a process of refinement for me. The process isn't pleasant and can be real uncomfortable at times. I want it to move faster than it is. I know when it's completed that I'll be a better witness for Jesus.

I awoke one morning with these words in my head: *To rush the process would be to ruin the process.*

I will wait, watch, listen, and pray to be ready when the process is complete in His timing.

OLD STORIES: NOAH

January 23, 2011

On the first of the year, I started a new 365-day Bible reading plan. As you would expect, it starts with the beginning and finishes at the end of the Bible. So there I was starting in Genesis reading the old Bible stories that I've heard since I was knee high to a grasshopper. I've heard or read these stories so many times, I was wondering if I could really learn anything new. It didn't take long for God to reach down and cuff me one with a resounding, "Yes!"

I was reading the story of Noah and the ark and how God had told Noah that He was going to destroy all living things on the face of the earth. God gave Noah instructions on how to build the ark and how many of each type of animal was to be brought on the ark. Then tucked in the story was this short verse:

Noah did according to all that the LORD had commanded him.

—GENESIS 7:5

It would take Noah 120 years to build the ark, but he did everything just as God had commanded. That's a long-term commitment to God's plan. I have a hard time doing what God commands for just a day or two. I've only been at this cancer-fighting thing for six months, and there are days that I get frustrated with the pace things are moving. Those are the days I have to remind myself that God has a plan, and I have to stick with it.

Once the waters began to recede, Noah began sending out birds to see if the land was dry. Finally, a dove returned with an olive branch and gave Noah assurance the land was dry. However, Noah didn't leave the ark. He waited for God to tell him it was time to leave the ark. I'm pretty sure that after spending 120 years building, living with all those animals and enduring rain for forty days and nights, I couldn't have waited to get out of there. That's another failing of mine: I don't enjoy waiting. Slowly, God is teaching me.

These past few weeks, there's been a consistent theme running through my life. From Noah to messages I've heard on television and radio, all of them have been about God's will in your life and waiting. Sometimes it feels like God is only working when I see things happening.

I'm beginning to learn that God is in the waiting too.

THE GREATEST MAN I HAVE EVER KNOWN

February 3, 2011

I still remember the assignments in grade school where we were instructed to write about the person who had had the biggest influence on our young lives. My first inclination was to write about my professional sports heroes; however, I really didn't know them and, in most instances, their character has not proven to be admirable. Looking back, I can find only one man who has passed the test of time.

I'm now fifty-one years old and have known the man I write about for all those years. During this time, he's certainly grown wiser, braver, more intelligent, and bigger than life itself. Without a doubt, he's the greatest man I've ever known.

He grew up on the family farm in West Virginia. He was the oldest of five children and had to bear all of the duties and responsibilities of being the big brother. The family worked this farm throughout the Great Depression. This period in his life shaped his attitudes concerning financial dealings and hard work.

After graduating from high school, he joined the U.S. Army Air Corps. He spent most of World War II in the States learning to maintain B-29 bombers and held the rank of technical sergeant. The flight crew he was in was sent to Okinawa the day the Japanese surrendered, saving them from making any bombing runs. Even though he didn't see any active duty, I'm amazed at the willingness of this man to make the ultimate sacrifice for his country.

He married my mom during the war. After he was released from the Air Corps, they moved to Oklahoma, where he got a job working at the post office. The family grew with six kids, and to support his family, he took a second job on the weekends, working in the body shop of a local car dealership.

I remember he always took great pride in the way he looked in his post office uniform. His trousers and shirts were always pressed, with his shoes and bill of his cap shined. He was a representative of the U.S. government. That's the way he went to work until he retired.

Dad and Mom had been married sixty years when she passed away. From what I've related here, this may seem like an ordinary life to most. He never achieved great financial success. He had to work hard for every penny he ever made. He never possessed any political clout, nor did he ever seek any. So what makes this man so great?

Together he and Mom raised six kids to be productive members of society. None of those kids ever became involved in drugs or spent any time in jail. All those children were taught to respect their elders and that to achieve something through hard work was something to be proud of. Although this family was never wealthy by worldly terms, they certainly never thought they were poor. The children were taught to be thankful for what they had and to always take care of their "needs" before worrying about the "wants." Many fathers have either taught or strived to teach their children these same lessons. In the minds of most, this doesn't qualify as greatness.

What makes this man different is that he's where I got my vision of what my heavenly Father is like. I know that, just like my Father above, my earthly dad had sometimes been disappointed in my actions, but he never stopped loving me. I know at times I wandered from the path my dad wished I would take, but he waited patiently for me to find my way back. Sure, there were times when I was spanked or otherwise corrected; however, it was done because he loved me too much to let me stray too far.

My dad taught me what it means to be a father and a husband. I will never know the number of times he went without so the family could have something it needed. He taught me that being a father and husband was sacrificing himself for the family. Family is everything.

The most important thing he taught me was to keep your faith and God first. I remember him studying his Bible every night. We were in church every Sunday, where he led the singing, taught Sunday school, and served as a deacon and elder. Every other week my dad would sit at the kitchen table and make out the checks to support the church or various missionaries around the world. He always made sure to give the tithe or more. Not only did he support the missionaries financially, but when they stopped in town for a conference, they even slept at our home. I'm confident that when my dad got to heaven, he met people from all over the world who are there because he cared enough to support all those missionaries.

Mom passed away in 2005. During her final days with us, Dad continued to teach me, not by his word, but by his actions. He taught me during those days about love—what it means to love another so deeply that, although in your heart you long to keep them with you, sometimes it's better to let them go.

Just ten months later, the ails of this world took their toll on his fragile body. Even as his body was beginning to fail him, he still taught me. This time he taught me to suffer with dignity.

I know that when Daddy closed his eyes on this earth, he opened them in heaven, and there to greet him was Mom. Now the two of them, together for sixty years here, will spend eternity together.

This is the man that I have come to see as great. Granted, as I was growing up, that wasn't always my opinion. Now that I'm married and have two boys of my own, I hope I can be the father to them that my dad was and still is to me.

Thanks, Daddy, for showing me the way. I'll see you in heaven.

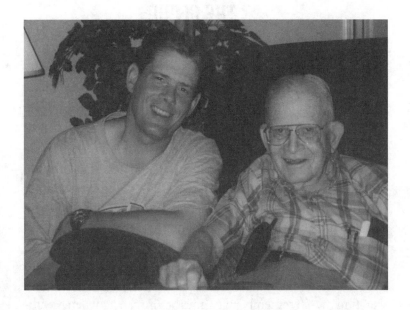

IN THE CLOUD

February 20, 2011

Looking back over these past few months, there have been times I'm certain the life I'm living isn't mine. There have been days that as soon as I wake up, a cloud descends on me. I spend the day going through the motions. I go to bed at night praying that when I awake the next morning, the cloud will lift, I'll find God's plan in all this, and the nightmare will cease. That hasn't happened yet.

Sometimes the cloud is of my own making. I can retreat into the cloud away from the doctors, nurses, and loud machines. I can find myself remembering times before cancer when breathing was easier, and there was no coughing to remind me. I'm finding that if I stay in my cloud too long, that's when the self-pity begins. My cloud can become dark and depressing.

Other times I think that the cloud is from God. These are the days I have to depend on Him to get me through the day. I believe He's trying to teach me to increase my dependence on Him. That doesn't make this any easier, but it helps to know that when the fatigue sets in, He's there to carry me.

One thing I've continued to struggle with is worshiping God in all this. I know that if these clouds would lift, then I'll be able to worship God for what He's done. But I've been reminded that isn't always how it works. When God gave Moses the instructions concerning the temple in the final chapter of Exodus, then a cloud covered the Tent of Meeting. This was to be a sign that

God was there, and the people were to stay and worship God in that place.

On occasion, I've wondered where God has gone.

Now I know He has always been right here in the cloud with me.

A DAD, A SON, AND HIS BIKES

February 26, 2011

I may have mentioned once or twice that Chad and Shane are into bicycles. Well, not "into" bicycles—they practically live to ride bikes. Chad got into cycling because of a friend; Shane got into cycling because of Chad. Both of them possess a natural talent for racing bikes, but they're different types of riders. Chad is a long-distance racer, and Shane is a sprinter. Chad started his serious racing after he went to college; Shane started racing his junior year in high school, and I drove him to all of his high school races. I still enjoy thinking about the great memories built during that time shared.

In November of his junior year, there was a mountain bike endurance race held at Erwin Park in McKinney. Shane thought it was a good idea for him to enter the six-hour division and asked if I would be his race support. I agreed, not realizing it would also be a six-hour endurance test for me. My job was to carry a backpack full of water, Gatorade, and snacks for him during the race. The morning of the race was clear and bitter cold. I was to be in one of two clearings at the park. As he passed in one clearing, he'd tell me what he wanted. I'd then run to the other clearing and have it ready for him when he got there. We did this for six hours, and we made a good team. When he crossed the finish line for the last time, we were both proud of what he accomplished. He won.

Early in the spring of 2008, Shane was in desperate need of a new road bike. One Saturday, I asked him if he wanted to go look at bikes to see what they cost. Off we went to the first bike shop, but he didn't find anything there that he liked. We headed for a much larger bicycle shop that offered a better selection. He looked around for a bit before finding a red-and-white Specialized bike that he liked. We talked to the sales guy for a bit about the bike, and then I looked at Shane.

"Is that the one you want?" I asked.

He had a great "you are kidding" look on his face. Thirty minutes later we were loading up his new bike.

Shane didn't get to race much in 2008 because it conflicted with high school baseball, but he decided that during his senior year, he wanted to race bikes instead of play baseball. Shane and I spent the spring of his senior year loading up his bike and driving all across Texas so he could race. His main goal was to win the Texas High School Racing League. I had a lot of fun watching him race. Each race he got stronger. When he decided it was time to go for the win, he would just ride off from the other racers. That red-and-white bike carried him to a lot of wins that spring. Finally, he brought home the overall first-place trophy from the state championship in Amarillo.

Two weeks ago, Shane called to let me know he had crashed in a race. The impact was so hard, it had broken the frame on his bike. Thankfully, Shane only suffered sprained wrists, but the bike was history. Later that night as I thought about that bike, I began to tear up a little. I thought of all of the places we had taken that bike together. It was like an old friend was gone, leaving only memories behind. That bike had carried Shane from a beginning "Category 4" racer to an experienced "Category 1" and into his second year of collegiate racing. I know it may be silly to think that way about a bike, but it took Shane a long way and held a lot of memories for both of us.

Reflecting about buying the bike and the time spent with Shane going to races, I have to say that red-and-white bike was, undoubtedly, the best investment I ever made.

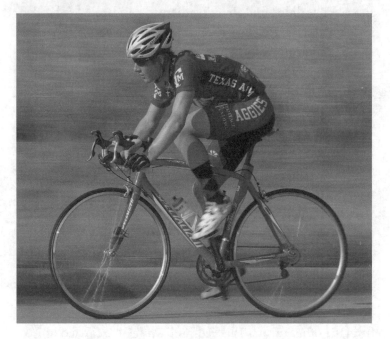

PRAYERS

March 8, 2011

I've never been very good at praying. I start, then lose my focus, and my mind begins to wander. Soon I forget what I am praying about, get frustrated, and give up. During radiation treatment, I remembered hearing a minister say that if you don't know what to pray for, then pray the Bible. I thought I could surely handle that. I read the psalms, underlined verses that ministered to me, and used them as my morning prayers. I read ten psalms a day for fifteen days, underlining and praying Scripture back to God. After fifteen days, I felt these had to have been some of the most heartfelt, effective prayers of my life and decided I'd start over and do them again. I've continued doing this. I'm still amazed how the right verses come up on the days I need them most.

On day fifteen, when I was at my lowest point physically, I read the very last verse.

Let everything that has breath praise the LORD. Praise the LORD!

—PSALM 150:6

That's a tough pill to swallow for a lung cancer patient. But I still had breath, so I praised the Lord.

The days leading up to the tests and treatments are the most anxious. There seem to always be a lot of what-ifs running through my mind. Every time I get worried, psalms come up about God calming a situation. Because I've always had the vision that this cancer battle was like being in a boat tossed by the waves, these verses touched me the most.

For He spoke and raised up a stormy wind, which lifted up the waves of the sea. They rose up to the heavens, they went down to the depths; their soul melted away in their misery. They reeled and staggered like a drunken man, and were at their wits' end. Then they cried to the LORD in their trouble, and He brought them out of their distresses. He caused the storm to be still, so that the waves of the sea were hushed.
—PSALM 107:25–29

Finally, after seven months, we heard the news we'd been waiting for. The cancer hasn't spread to any new sites. The previous active sites are now either inactive or decreased in activity. The primary lung tumor has shrunk by half and is possibly dead!

The next morning, Psalm 81 was the first for my daily prayer. It evoked memories of the distant thunderous sounds of the MRI machines we heard while walking the halls of MD Anderson. Here's what I had underlined some three months ago:

Sing for joy to God our strength; shout joyfully to the God of Jacob. . . . "You called in trouble and I rescued you; I answered you in the hiding place of thunder."
—PSALM 81:1, 7

I can't add anything to that but "Amen!"

A LIFE SENTENCE

March 20, 2011

This is a post I've been putting off for several days. I'm afraid people will take what I'm about to write about as bragging or that I think I have it all figured out. I hope you believe that I've prayed about what to write. Please read and accept this entry in the spirit it is intended. Only God can make you see things the way I see them now.

I've heard multiple times from friends, co-workers, family, doctors, and nurses about what a great positive attitude I have. It's the same attitude I've had my whole life. One co-worker told me she's glad to see that cancer hasn't changed my attitude like with other cancer sufferers. I told her there was enough negativity in the world without me adding to it.

What has helped me the most is that I don't see cancer as a death sentence. I see it as a life sentence. I firmly believe that God's will is for me to be completely healed from cancer and that it will never return. When that happens, I will live every day with gratitude for that momentous event, loving my family, enjoying the days with them, and I will continue to worship Jesus.

There are some people who will ask, "What if God's will is for you not to be healed?"

If the time should come that cancer takes my earthly body, I am certain that my belief in Jesus Christ means that when I take my last breath on earth, I will then take my first breath in heaven. I will then have two good lungs, and there will be no more pain. I will see my family and friends who have gone before me, and I will continue to worship Jesus.

Either way, I still live!

MORE THAN I CAN HANDLE

March 23, 2011

"Remember, God never gives you more than you can handle."
You've likely heard someone say that or possibly even said it yourself. I've had people repeat it to me these past several months. The majority of them have been Christians offering me words of encouragement. If you're one of those people that have used this phrase, then I may offend you, because I don't think it's true.

If God doesn't give me more than I can handle, then why do I have cancer? Just ask DeLayne—I'm an absolute wimp when it comes to just having a cold. I don't like going to the doctor, much less having needles inserted in my hand and arms for blood draws and IVs. If DeLayne weren't along to keep the ever-changing schedule straight and take care of all the insurance paperwork, I would be in one big mess. Cancer is more than I can handle.

If God doesn't give me more than I can handle, then what has been the role of my friends and family who have hoisted us on their shoulders while on their knees in prayer? If I could handle this on my own, there wouldn't be any need for these numerous people who have rallied around us to offer us support and food at home and in Houston. No, I can't handle cancer by myself.

If God doesn't give me more than I can handle, then what role is there for Jesus? If I were able to fix this on my own, exactly when would I learn to depend on Him? Jesus, Himself, said,

"Come to Me, all who are weary and heavy-laden, and I will give you rest" (Matthew 11:28). I'm so thankful for that invitation. There are days that cancer and all that goes with it overwhelms me. No, I *cannot* handle cancer by myself.

Another saying I have heard is, "If God brings you to it, He will bring you through it."

I've changed that to, "If God brings you to it, He can carry you through it."

No, I can't handle cancer by myself, but I don't have to.

SIN AND LOVE HELD HIM THERE

April 19, 2011

Jesus had led them back to the garden. Whenever He wanted to be alone and pray, this is where He would go. They had just finished the Passover meal, and He had washed their feet. There had been an exchange between Him and Judas; Judas had run from the room and hadn't returned.

Now Jesus and the remaining eleven had returned to the garden. Eight of the disciples had stopped to rest. Peter, James, and John went on ahead with Jesus. Jesus told them to watch and pray and then went on to pray by Himself. A short while later, Jesus returned to find them sleeping. He encouraged them, again, to watch and pray. They could tell by the way Jesus looked and acted that He was in anguish. But they still couldn't stay awake. He returned, again, to find them sleeping. He woke them and told them that His time was at hand.

They could see the mob coming up the hill. Judas was leading the mob, and Jesus went out to meet them. Judas stepped forward and kissed Jesus on the cheek. The mob moved to arrest Jesus. Peter leaped forward to defend Jesus and pulled his knife, slicing off the ear of a servant. Jesus admonished Peter to put away his knife. He didn't need Peter to defend Him. If He wanted to, He could call down the angels in heaven, and they would lay waste to the mob. But that wasn't His plan. Jesus was led away by the mob to be tried.

Jesus didn't defend Himself at the trial. He was led from place to place, beaten multiple times, mocked, and spat upon. Still, no retaliation would come from Him. He was made to carry His own cross until His strength was gone. The Roman solders nailed His hands and feet to the cross. The taunting continued as they gambled for His clothes. Look at Him there, hanging on that cross. Blood pouring down His face from the crown of thorns pressed into His head. His body bloodied and bruised from the beatings. His shoulders dislocated and His legs straining to keep his body upright, gasping for air. Jesus Christ was experiencing complete and total humiliation.

Would He call the angels now? The angels had to be ready, incensed by the treatment of God Almighty by a world that didn't deserve Him. They could have come and taken Him back to heaven where He belonged. No. He wouldn't call on the angels in heaven. He stayed there on that cross. Why? What held Him on the cross? The soldiers? No. The nails? No. None of these kept Him hanging on the cross. It was the sin of the world—your sin, my sin—and His love for us that kept Him there.

Isn't it amazing that, while hanging there, Jesus Christ could see my face and know the only way I could enter heaven was for Him to die on that cross, and He chose to do it anyway?

RIGHT PEOPLE, RIGHT PLACE, RIGHT TIME

April 26, 2011

About one year ago, my symptoms began to appear. We had no idea then what type of journey we were beginning. It would take another three months before we would have the diagnosis. Looking back over the past year, it's obvious God has placed each stepping-stone in our pathway and securely placed our feet on each stone along the way. Early on, I prayed God would place the right people in the right place at the right time to help us deal with cancer. God has been faithful to answer that prayer, and we have experienced an amazing journey.

One of the first people that God sent my way was a dog. I mean a *real* dog. At our house, dogs are people too. Pepper came along the morning after I was told I had stage IV lung cancer. I needed something to laugh about, and there came Pepper bouncing into the water fountain. I never thought watching a dog try to catch water as it spurted from a fountain could supply such joy. Even today, I still smile when I think about Pepper.

Another person that God used was my Gamma Knife nurse. She escorted me all morning and pushed me all over the hospital. She provided me with information about what was happening and what the next step would be. She seemed to sense that I needed information and that silence wasn't good for me. During our talks, I learned she isn't a Christian and no longer practices the faith she grew up in. She's now on my prayer list.

I was admitted to the hospital just three days before I was to have a port placed in my chest with chemo scheduled the following day. An oncologist finally recognized I had postobstructive pneumonia. In my condition, chemo could have killed me. My entire treatment plan was changed immediately. This doctor also had me tested for the rare mutation it turned out that I have.

When I was admitted to the hospital after my third chemo treatment, God sent another nurse to minister to me in a special way. After seeing me reading my Bible, she shared with me a message she had seen on television that day about healing. She looked at me and asked if I had faith that I would be healed. When I replied, "Yes," she walked over to my bedside and placed her hands on my chest and then prayed for my complete healing. I doubt they teach that in nursing school.

I was treated to a day of tests and scans to prepare me for the clinical trial, including a bone scan. It was my first bone scan, and I was concerned because it seemed after every new test was done, cancer was found somewhere else. After completing the bone scan, I went for blood work and an EKG. In the EKG room, I noticed a Bible on the technician's desk. She asked if I believed in God. I replied, "Yes," and with my permission, she started a song on her computer. I don't recall the title of the song, but it was about how great God is. I was reminded that no matter the outcome of the scan, God wouldn't be surprised and had the situation under His control.

God has taught me over the past year that He will answer prayers at a time, place, and way of His choosing. I look at people differently now knowing that God has placed each one of them in my path for His purposes. In addition to doctors, nurses, and technicians, there have been friends and family members who just seemed to know when I needed a phone call, text, or an email for encouragement. Others have brought us food and nourished us both physically and spiritually. We'll never be able to thank them enough for standing with us during this time.

CHASING DREAMS

May 9, 2011

We parents have dreams for our children that we begin building the day they are born. The dreams typically include doing well in school, going on to college, graduating, and starting a career. Somewhere along the way, they'll meet the right person and get married. Then one day, we realize the dreams we have for our children are essentially the lives we have lived. There comes a day when our dreams and our children's dreams no longer travel the same path or even intersect. Although we've strived to prepare them to leave the nest, they have suddenly climbed out on the branch by themselves before we realize it, ready to spread their wings and take the leap on their own.

That's how it's been with Chad. He was doing pretty well living my own dream for him and was within months of graduating from college with his mechanical engineering degree. A job was pretty much lined up, but instead, he had his own dreams to chase.

One afternoon last October, he called to tell me there were a couple of elite amateur bike teams that had shown an interest in him. After mulling it over, he had consulted with one of his teammates. Both teams seemed like good opportunities. During the call, I sensed there was something he wanted to ask me, but he never did.

While I lay in bed that night, I pondered what Chad hadn't asked. I believed he wanted to know how I felt about his pursuing cycling after graduation. I had mixed emotions about it all. I hated to see him walk away from a good job, but I also wanted to see him pursue something he has a passion for. I woke up the next morning with the answer. I didn't want Chad to ever have to wonder, *What if?*

I called him later that day and told him that now was the time for him to go for it. I explained I did not want him to grow up and find himself in my same situation. I was fifty years old with cancer and wondering, *Would I ever get to do the things I had put off for so long?* Cancer has taught me to pursue the dreams while they're fresh.

Chad now lives in Colorado and is living his dream by criss-crossing the country racing his bike while chasing another dream, that of becoming a professional cyclist.

I have no doubt he will make it.

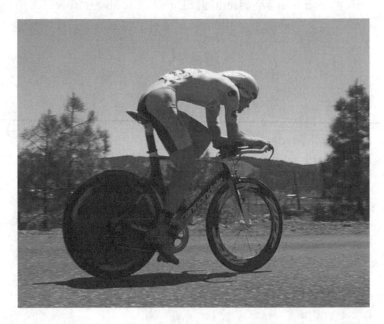

WET FEET

May 23, 2011

Thursday, May 26, will be my twelve-week checkup for the clinical trial medicine. It's hard to believe that twelve weeks have passed already. I'm somewhat excited about this visit because I've read reports that indicate twelve weeks is when they've seen significant changes in tumors. One patient saw his tumors completely disappear at this point. As is my habit, I've begun to prepare myself mentally and spiritually for my checkup next week.

The story of Exodus has been on my mind the past few days. God had parted the Red Sea for the Israelites to escape Egypt and Pharaoh's army. God provided for their every need on their journey through the desert for forty years. However, they still had doubts and questioned God. I'm sure they had to be asking, *How much longer can this go on? When will we be allowed to enter the promised land?*

Although it hasn't quite been a year since I was diagnosed, I have found myself comparing my journey to that in the exodus. God has parted the waters countless times to give me safe passage through troubled waters. He has met my every need in ways I've never imagined. However, I've been asking, *Will next week be when I enter into the promised land of complete healing?*

To finally enter the promised land, the Israelites had to cross the Jordan River. Only this time God required some action from the people. The priests were to carry the ark of the covenant into the Jordan. Once all of the priests had entered the river, the water would stop. The people would cross on dry land.

God has used the story of Exodus and entering the promised land to teach me that He will lead you through the wilderness. But to get from where you are to where God desires you to be, you have to be willing to get your feet wet.

LIMITS

May 31, 2011

On May 18, I came home from work, changed clothes, and went out for my usual bike ride. I had completed a couple of laps around the neighborhood and realized my breathing seemed to come with more ease. I continued and, out of nowhere, I heard that same voice that had told me I was in for a long, hard battle. This time the message was, *The tumor is gone.* A week later, with those words echoing in my head, I once again slid into the machine for my CT scan.

The next morning, we waited in the examination room for my entourage. In the clinical trial, I now see four people at each appointment: two research assistants, the physician's assistant, and the doctor. I jokingly call them my entourage. With the suspense building, finally, one of the research assistants came in to pick up my empty medicine bottles and the research survey. He then handed us the reports from radiology for the x-ray and CT scan. He informed us that they were still waiting on the MRI report from that same morning. He left DeLayne and me to read the reports. We noticed mention of the fluid and scar tissue in my lung, but nowhere did we read mention of the lung tumor. These were the first reports that did not specifically mention the presence or the size of the mass in my lung. Could the tumor really be gone?

Finally, all of the medical team except the doctor entered the examining room. The physician's assistant told us that all the reports looked great. She informed us that there was "no evidence of disease" (NED) and asked if we had any questions. I, of course, asked if the absence of the tumor in the reports meant the tumor was gone. She explained that sometimes the radiologist doesn't mention the tumor and that NED doesn't necessarily mean the tumor is gone. Instead, it just means there's no evidence of "active" cancer and that this is as good as it gets for lung cancer patients. The medical profession will never say a lung cancer patient is cured or in remission.

After a few minutes, my doctor entered the exam room. He informed us that the test results and the way I'm feeling were all very encouraging. I repeated the question about the tumor. He explained that due to the damage done to my lung from the radiation treatments and cancer, it was very difficult to tell if the tumor was still present. This led us to ask if my lung would ever recover.

He replied, "No. Performing radiation on any portion of the lung is essentially like removing that portion of the lung."

I did not expect to hear those words from the doctor. Nonetheless, I still believe I'll be completely healed, which includes my lung returning to fully functioning. After a few days of contemplation, my interpretation of what the doctor said became that we've determined the limits of what medicine can do for me. From here on, all improvements to my lung will be 100 percent miracles from God.

In Mark 3:1–5, Jesus healed a man with a withered hand in the synagogue. This story has, naturally, been on my mind. I'm very thankful and blessed by what God has done for me this past year, and if He can heal a withered hand, He can certainly heal my lung.

While we may have reached the limits of medicine, there's no limit to what God can do.

THINGS CANCER HAS TAUGHT ME

June 16, 2011

I remember when I was first diagnosed, I thought I shouldn't have lung cancer. Even one of the doctors agreed: "You shouldn't have this, but you do." I also remember praying that God would use this as an opportunity for us to teach others about lung cancer and present us with those openings. I could share that if I could have lung cancer, then anyone could develop lung cancer. Little did I know at the time what cancer would teach *me*.

One thing I've learned is to laugh every day. When you think you're tired of laughing, laugh some more. There have been times that if I hadn't laughed, I would have cried. The thing that has surprised me is how many openings the medical staff provided me for a joke. They get accustomed to saying the same things and aren't prepared for someone like me.

For instance, at one of my blood specimen collections, the tech said, "Today we need to get urine on you." I replied, "How about I put it in a cup?"

Then there was the day I was being prepped for an MRI. I lost count of the number of times I was asked if there was any metal in my body. One tech was being very serious with questioning and then asked, "Is there any metal in your body?" I replied, "Only if the aliens left something." She really tried to not laugh but finally gave up.

I've learned to cherish every moment of every day. Life has a different pace now. Gone is the rushing. I find myself taking time to look about and really see what is going on. Why do we race from place to place? Take time to enjoy where you are and who you are with. You will never have that moment in time again.

I have always believed in the Bible, but this experience has taught me the Bible is more than just words on paper. The Bible is the very living, breathing Word of God. I've witnessed the Scriptures come alive daily.

One thing that has surprised me is the epiphany that everyone has a "cancer" in their life. Mine is physical, but others may be dealing with porn, gambling, alcohol, issues at work, financial stressors, or problems with a child or spouse. Everybody has something that, given time, can and will grow. Like cancer, if left untreated, it will take your life.

The great thing is that we have One who sits at the right hand of God ready to help us. I'm thankful that He's there.

THE WIND AT MY BACK

June 21, 2011

The weather has turned hot here in North Texas. Once again, we seemed to have jumped from winter directly into summer. Winds gusting out of the south have the temperatures already hitting 100 degrees. To avoid riding in a convection oven, I am riding after dinner and early on Saturday morning.

Last Saturday morning I was getting ready for my ride and could hear the wind blowing and see the tree tops swaying. I began to ride and could feel a gale blustering against me as I headed out of the neighborhood. I was greeted with a strong blast as I turned south. *This won't be a fun ride.* The first half of the ride, I struggled up every little hill and fought the wind with every turn. I knew I'd been struggling when I looked at my speedometer that read only "12 mph." Then I saw the arrow moving up, indicating my average speed was increasing.

I finally made the turn to head back north, and I could feel the wind at my back, pushing me along. Picking up some speed, I reached for the shifter with my left hand and moved it to the right. The chain moved to the big ring, and I began to pedal harder. Then, suddenly, they were back. My legs and my breathing were in my precancer rhythm. I started pushing the pedals harder as I shifted through the gears with my right hand. Picking up speed, I glanced at the speedometer: "20 mph, 22 mph . . ." How long and how hard could I push it?

Then I realized this morning's ride was a perfect analogy for my last year. I had been riding against the wind and, at times, struggling to get over the hills. Now I'm riding with the wind at my back, pushing hard, and getting back into rhythm.

I looked back down just in time to see "25 mph." When I looked up, I realized I was close to the intersection where I would make a right turn to head back home. As I pedaled through the turn, I looked down to see "23 mph" displayed. With a smile on my face, I yelled at the cancer, "You will not win!"

After a drink of cool water, I began pushing the pedals toward home, laughing. It's good to feel the wind at my back.

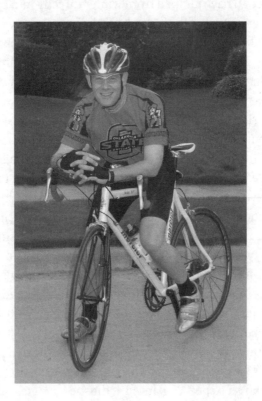

ONE MORE HILL

July 9, 2011

There are times when I ride that I try to see how fast I can go and other times to make it a test of endurance. I was getting tired of riding just ten miles. Today, I decided to determine how far I had come by seeing how far I could go.

In case I'm not feeling up to a long ride, I intentionally plan my routes to include places to turn around and head back home. This morning, I found myself bypassing the turnoffs and riding on roads that I haven't ridden in a year. By the time I hit the nine-mile mark, I was committed. I was also out of gas. I stopped on a side street to drink some water and catch my breath, and I was trying to decide whether to call DeLayne to come get me. But I decided that if I gave up now, cancer would win one. I determined that if it took me all day to finish the ride, then that's what I would do. Resolute, I clipped my feet back on the pedals and continued my ride.

At mile fifteen, I had reached the next to last intersection on the home stretch. After stopping for the red light, I looked up, and there staring at me, barely a half mile away, was one more hill to climb. I hate this hill! I have to climb this hill on every ride, and it's always a struggle. I could hear it taunting me this morning: *You don't have the legs left today.* The light turned green, and the first few pedal strokes felt as if I was riding in wet concrete. I reached the start of the hill and had to grit my teeth. It took every bit of what I had left to get up and over that hill. Finally, I was coasting toward home.

As I rode up to our front walk, the odometer clicked to seventeen miles—half of what I used to do on Saturdays but seven miles more than usual. I was happy with the effort and did a very sad and weak happy dance.

Once again, I'd proven to myself that I may have cancer, but cancer doesn't have me.

DOUBTS

July 26, 2011

"You may get cancer out of your body, but you will never get cancer out of your mind."

A friend shared that statement with me at one of the very first cancer encouragement groups we attended. Truer words have never been spoken.

I can scarcely remember a time in the last year that I doubted I would beat cancer. However, the past week has been a constant battle on many fronts. It has been a stark reminder that this is a physical battle as well as a spiritual and mental battle. We were disheartened to learn of our circle of friends being impacted by cancer. There was yet another new cancer diagnosis, two friends who are having complications with their treatments, and another friend losing his battle with cancer. Although I currently have no evidence of disease, cancer has been relentlessly attacking every day, creating doubts and causing me to lose my focus.

In the middle of this beatdown, my morning Bible reading took me to the story of Peter walking on the water with Jesus. Peter was doing fine until he noticed the wind. Then he began to sink.

All the news this past week caused me to notice the wind. I took my focus off Jesus—the very One who has gotten me through the past year. Jesus will never leave me nor forsake me. I'm thankful that when I begin to sink, He's there to grab my hand too.

STANDING ON THE PEDALS

September 3, 2011

I haven't written much lately. I confess that I have not felt like writing because of the frustratingly slow progress I've been making. It came to a head last Saturday when I drove up to the north side of McKinney. On the way, I saw people riding on the hills that I used to ride on. With each passing rider, I grew more frustrated that I was unable to ride like they were. I was sitting at a stop light, and I heard cancer throw down the challenge, *You can't do that anymore.* It was time to resume the battle.

This morning, I was up early and completed my quiet time reading. Then praying, I asked for God to provide me a good bike ride. I filled my bottles with water and Gatorade, readied my bike, and was out the door by 6:30. Riding out of the neighborhood, I turned north for the first time in over a year. Today, I was going to ride cancer into the pavement.

The morning air felt cool on my arms. Before long, I had reached the first downhill section, and I could hear the air rushing by my ears. It's been too long since I've heard that sound. I was able to make it up the next hill with minimal effort, and I started another descent. Before I knew it, I had made it up and over the three hills and was on my way to north McKinney. However, I knew that to get home, I'd have to ride back over these same hills. The way home is the hard part.

At mile ten, there they were: the three hills. I enjoyed them on the way out, but now I would need to defeat them with tired legs. But this was the reason I chose this route. I had to prove that I could meet this challenge. Slowly, I made my way up the first hill. At the top, I was passed by a rider who flew by me like I was going backward. As I made my way down the first hill, I sucked in as much air as I could and prepared to ascend the second hill. About halfway up the second hill, I had to stand up on the pedals. I took a few pedal strokes and then coasted. Then I repeated. I reached the top and began sucking in air again. I hoped for a long descent, but it was over quickly, and I started up the final hill—the worst one.

Halfway up, I was out of the saddle again and was back up on the pedals. After a few seconds, I had to sit back down to try and catch whatever breath I could. As I approached the top, I was standing on the pedals. This time, frustration and sheer determination provided the fuel I needed to get to the top, and I successfully met the challenge. Grateful to see a flat section of road, I sang the Doxology.

Each day may bring a new challenge, but each day is a blessing.

PURPOSE: PART 1

October 4, 2011

I seriously want a do-over for the month of September. It's just been one thing after another. I don't ever remember continually hurting myself so much in one month.

The month started with accidentally kicking a kitchen chair. My little toe, largely forgotten, made a ninety-degree right turn and a really nasty sound. I was amazed at the pain generated by such a little digit. All the toes on my right foot turned black and blue from the injury, and it hurt to put any kind of shoe on.

Two weeks later, I was still slightly hobbled when we went to Hawaii. While enjoying the scenery at a waterfall, the sidewalk had a slight turn to the left, and my right foot landed half on and half off the sidewalk. In the blink of an eye, my ankle rolled, and I was on the ground. Thankfully, this time only my pride was injured, with DeLayne the sole witness of my gracefulness.

A couple of nights later I was returning to bed from what old guys have to do in the middle of the night. In the dark, I managed to catch my little toe on the nightstand and was yet again reminded of its presence. The next day, I was thankful for the wonderful invention known as flip-flops.

Days later, our vacation was over, and we loaded up and headed to the airport. After dropping our luggage at TSA, I felt a slight twinge in my back. As we headed to security, I picked up my camera backpack and slung it over my shoulder. I would swear someone shoved a knife in my back. By the time we arrived home in Texas, it hurt to lie down, stand up, sit down, or just breathe.

The next week we packed again and went for my checkup in Houston. The CT scan showed a slight inflammation in my left lung. The doctor asked if I had been sick lately or coughing more. "No, not really," I replied. He thought it was an infection and prescribed a round of antibiotics. The doctor probably doesn't realize he's a fortune teller, as the next afternoon, I had a scratchy throat and started coughing.

By the weekend, I was coughing and sneezing with a head and chest cold. Every time I sneezed, my back hurt a little bit more. By Sunday morning, I was absolutely miserable, and about all I could do was sit in the recliner.

During times like these, I grow frustrated and start asking God questions I don't expect Him to answer: *What is the purpose of all of this?* and, *What is the purpose for my having cancer?*

But suddenly, there it was, and I was surprised at how simple the answer was. I thought if I were to receive an answer, it would be something really deep and astounding. It wasn't. Only six simple words flashed through my head.

So that God will be glorified.

I'll pass on the do-over.

WHAT A VIEW

October 16, 2011

During our vacation in Hawaii, we visited the island of Kauai. One of the must-sees on the island is Waimea Canyon, which has been called the Grand Canyon of Hawaii.

There are two routes to drive up Waimea Canyon, and one way is more scenic than the other. The reason it's more scenic is because it starts at sea level, climbs to over 5,000 feet, and skirts the canyon rim. DeLayne has never done well on these kinds of roads, but she wanted to take the scenic route anyway. The road is a narrow two-lane road that twists and turns its way up the mountain. There are steep climbs followed by rapid descents, blind corners followed by hairpin turns. She white-knuckled it all the way up. I'm sure she left finger impressions in the armrest and dashboard. She held my water bottle some of the time, and when we got out of the car, I discovered it was crushed from her squeezing it too hard. We still aren't sure if the drive is really all that scenic. DeLayne wouldn't look, and I wasn't allowed to look after being admonished multiple times to just watch the road.

After enduring all the ups and down and twists and turns, we reached the end of the canyon road. We had to climb a few stairs but were finally treated to a view of God's handiwork.

This trip makes me realize that someday we will come to the end of the road on this journey. We'll look back down the road we've been on and see all of the steep climbs, rapid descents, blind corners, and hairpin turns. We'll see all that God has done and His handiwork in our lives. We will say, "What a view!"

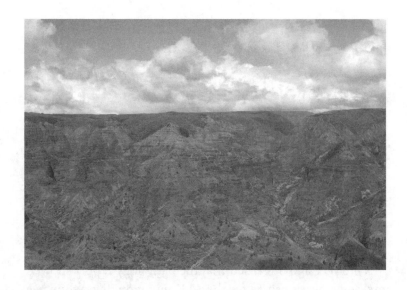

B-52

November 17, 2011

Well, here I am. I've made it to my fifty-second birthday—a
birthday that, except for the grace of God, the odds were
firmly against me seeing. One year ago, I had taken to sleeping
on the couch. After completing fifteen radiation treatments,
my right side and back hurt so much I had to prop myself up
on my left side to get any sleep.

One year ago, I learned that the pathology report showed
my cancer was positive for the ALK mutation. Everything we
did from then on was targeted to get me into a clinical trial for
a new medicine to treat ALK lung cancer. I was given a month
to recover from radiation and then started my first round of
required chemo treatments. Two months later, I was accepted
into the clinical trial. Twelve weeks after that, we received the
first report of no evidence of disease.

Over the past year, I've lost count of the number of people
I know who've lost their battles to beat cancer. But here I am,
muddling along and still kicking. There's no road map for this
quest to beat cancer. It's a day-by-day, step-by-step odyssey. I've
learned to trust God to place my feet on solid ground. The past
year has been as much an emotional struggle as a physical struggle. I've seen parts of my life erode away as if giant waves were
hitting a beach and sweeping the sand out to sea. At one time,
I prayed God would show me the unimportant parts of my life
and remove them. Is He answering that prayer?

This past year, I've developed a real appreciation for what Jesus did for me on the cross. There have been moments when every breath seemed to be a struggle. After fracturing three vertebrae in my back, it seemed like every bone in my body ached—and I wasn't nailed to a cross. The discomfort that I've experienced doesn't compare to the pain and suffering that Jesus experienced on my behalf. The day that Jesus was beaten and hung on a cross, He provided a way for my sins to be forgiven and for me to be healed.

Thank you, Jesus!

A BROKEN VESSEL

January 7, 2012

Broken. That's what I am—broken. I can't remember at any point in my life being as broken as I am right now. I told one of the doctors that it's like all my dominoes were in a line, and someone walked up and pushed the first one. Now I'm powerless to stop them. Since mid-September, there's been one health issue after another. They have finally taken their toll.

Physically, I'm exhausted. I'm not sure there's any part of my body that's working as it should. When it does work, it hurts. Just sitting up to eat or taking a short walk wears me out. Rolling over in bed takes tremendous effort. I try to not take many of the pain meds prescribed for me, but sometimes they're the only answer.

Emotionally, I find myself becoming more disconnected each day. The doctor from Care Support told me it's okay to cry and would probably be good for me. I just thought, *Dude, if I could, I would.* I feel like I have no control, and all the emotion has been sucked out of me.

Mentally, I'm fatigued. I feel like I have pulled all-nighters for finals for the past week. Putting two thoughts together is becoming a real challenge. I do my best to just focus on each day and what it will take to get through it. With the string of bad days that I've had, it's hard to think of better days coming.

Spiritually, I've been drained. This is the area that most disturbs me. I try to read my Bible, but I just can't muster the desire. I try to pray, but all that will come out is, "God, please fix something!" Early one morning, I was lying in bed, pleading with God to show me some mercy. Suddenly, I realized the song "It is Well with My Soul" was playing in my head. I got mad and told God that under no circumstances was any of this well with my soul. Then I tried to recall some memory verses. The only verse that would come to mind was "MY GOD, MY GOD, WHY HAVE YOU FORSAKEN ME?" (Matthew 27:46). That pretty well summed up my feelings at that moment.

I still believe God is here, and He's working. I just wish I could feel Him more. I still believe something good will come from all of this. I just wish I could see it. I still believe that God is and will be glorified in all of this. I just wish He would get some glory somewhere else for a while.

Can God still use a broken vessel like me? I've read before that God saves His greatest work for His vessels after they've been broken and He's put them back together. I guess we'll see how He puts this one back together.

THE PATHWAY BACK

January 22, 2012

After posting "A Broken Vessel," I was pretty well spent. I was uncertain as to how I would recover from all that had happened the previous week. I couldn't formulate a plan in my head and wasn't real impressed with where God's plan had me. It became evident that even though I wasn't particularly interested in spending time with God, He still wanted to spend time with me.

The next morning, I turned on the TV and, out of habit, looked for Dr. Charles Stanley's show. I found him and was shocked to hear that day's message was about challenges to our faith. When he said all of us face failures in our faith sometimes, I about yelled, "Preach on, Brother!" He went on to make the point that God uses these tests as a means to increase and stretch our faith. I began to realize I was being stretched, and it wasn't very comfortable.

After Dr. Stanley finished, I flipped a few more channels and heard another familiar voice. I had stumbled onto Dr. David Jeremiah's broadcast. His message that day was on fighting discouragement. *Really?* In the course of his message, he said all Christians will become discouraged. The only way to overcome deep discouragement is to read the Bible. Sometimes you'll be so discouraged that you'll have to force-feed yourself. He said you'll have to pray that God gives you verses of encouragement and that He sends you some encouragers.

So on Sunday afternoon, I humbled myself and asked God to forgive me for my bad attitude. I asked for Him to give me some verses of encouragement and to send people to encourage me. When I opened my Bible, God provided verses that, once again, established that He was, is, and will forever be in control. He knows my situation better than I do. I simply have to trust His direction.

That evening, my sister called to encourage me and lift my spirits. Then I started receiving emails and comments on my blog. People were thanking me for being honest about my battle, and they told me they'd be praying for me. Two days later, a woman I've never met left a comment for me about how my latest blog entry had helped her and her mother understand what another family member was going through. Even in my brokenness, God was still building.

These last two weeks, I've still had to force-feed myself some days. But at least I'm now on the pathway back.

WRESTLING WITH SATAN

January 30, 2012

During the previous two weeks, I started to spiritually find my way back and physically improve. I was tired of walking around the block and started walking the mile around the neighborhood. My breathing exercises showed real improvement.

I hadn't been able to attend church for several weeks. After this last stint in the hospital, I've been afraid of being in large groups of people, especially during the peak flu season. However, I knew I needed to be back in the body for worship.

After I got up Sunday morning and had breakfast, I did my first round of breathing exercises and saw the best early-morning results yet. I thought that was a good sign to start getting ready for church. However, after taking my shower, I noticed I was extremely short of breath. I also noticed my back was beginning to hurt worse. I started to doubt I'd be able to get out of the house. Sitting on the bed trying to catch my breath, I asked why, all of a sudden, this was such a battle.

That's when I heard my little voice say, *Satan doesn't want you in church.* Moving a little slower but with more determination, I continued to get ready for church. I could tell the wrestling match wasn't going to end.

After parking at church, we had a couple of hundred yards to walk to the entrance. The closer we got, the harder each step became. This was a much shorter walk than I've been doing, but, with each of the final few steps, I was saying, "Help me, Jesus."

Once I was in the church, I noticed that I was breathing hard, but my feet and legs felt lighter. I was able to make my way into the sanctuary, sit down, and begin catching my breath. I had made it to church.

After the service, I knew why Satan wrestled with me every step to church. Once again, the service was filled with hymns that contained words I needed to hear. The sermon was from Psalm 139 about how God had put me together. He knew the plans He had for me and that only He knew the number of my days. Satan didn't want me to be encouraged. He doesn't want me back in the game. But, thanks to Jesus, Satan has lost another match.

THE NEXT STEP

February 12, 2012

Have you ever had the feeling God wanted you to do something, but you just didn't feel like doing it? I've had that feeling the last couple of months. With everything else I've had to deal with, I just couldn't believe God was asking me to take the next step now. I was just being disobedient because I didn't feel well, and it involves doing something that I'm not comfortable with.

I've been feeling for the past couple of months that God wants me to go out and give my testimony. Writing this blog is one way to testify, but He has impressed upon me that reading about miracles is not enough. People also need to see and hear from the miracle. Today, I can relate to Moses. God wanted Moses to go to Pharaoh and lead His people out of Egypt. Moses' response was, "God, I am slow of speech and just not good at that."

People who know me understand that I avoid the spotlight, particularly speaking to a group. On occasion, I have forced myself to public speaking, but it pushes my comfort zone.

Like Moses, I am just going to trust God to provide the words, directions, and opportunities to present His message.

THE POTTER AND HIS CLAY

March 7, 2012

When I would sing the first stanza from the old hymn "Have Thine Own Way, Lord," I thought the verse had a gentle sentiment: Mold me and make me. I envisioned the gentle hand of the potter forming the clay as it spun on the wheel, knowing that any wrong moves would crumple the clay into a shapeless heap on the wheel. Until I saw a pottery demonstration.

Many years ago, we went to Eureka Springs to see *The Great Passion Play*. While we waited for the gates to open, we walked around and happened onto the pottery demonstration being given by the actor who would portray Jesus. We watched as he picked up a clump of clay and began forming it into a ball, gently rolling it around in his hands. Suddenly, he struck the clay with his fist and began pulling on it before forming a ball again. He repeated this a couple of times, explaining that he had to soften up the clay to make it compliant before he could create anything.

I've frequently thought about this scene and hymn the past months. Combining them, I have reached the conclusion that when Jesus is the potter, sometimes before He can use you, He has to make you useful. Yes, it may be uncomfortable and, at times, painful. But when He's done, you realize that, through the pain, He's made something wonderful and worthwhile.

TWENTY-ONE

April 14, 2012

In 1995, I was completing my MBA (Master of Business Administration), and I had spent too many evenings away from home and family. One evening, I didn't have any classwork and was able to pick the boys up from church. On the way home, the two boys were chattering away in the back seat, when Chad asked, "Daddy, how much longer do you have to go to school?"

"Just a few more weeks, why?"

Shane then piped up. "We just want our daddy back."

Ouch! I hadn't realized how my absences affected the boys.

Recently, that memory resurfaced while I was out for my walk. Two back surgeries to repair fractured vertebrae has meant that walking is one of the only forms of exercise I get these days. Sometimes during my walks, I think how much cancer has taken from my family. Pieces of my life have vanished, and life will never be the same. I'm slowly coming to grips with that. What is the most disturbing is that it doesn't seem right that my family is being put through this.

I remember the first time I saw my dad in a medical emergency. He was much older than I am now, and I was much older than our boys. I remember how my heart ached when I realized that he would be gone someday. It saddens me that, at this young age, my boys should have to consider such things and watch their daddy's life fade away.

Next week, that once little guy in the back seat turns twenty-one. I wish more than anything else that I could give him his daddy back.

PURPOSE: PART 2

May 8, 2012

We had spoken on the phone. He had just been diagnosed with stage IV lung cancer. The meeting had been arranged through mutual friends, and he wanted to know about my experience and treatment. I liked him, and we had things in common. He loved his family, he loved his wife, and he loved Jesus. He also was intent on beating lung cancer but knew the odds were against him. Just ten months later, his journey has come to an end. Cancer has taken another one.

Although I knew none of his treatments had been successful at slowing or stopping the cancer, the news of his passing caused me to reflect upon our similar circumstances. Both of us traveling the same road—one journey is finished and the other continues. God's plan and purpose is unique for each man. Yes, one man's plan and purpose is completed and the other marches on, but for what reason?

I struggle with what God's plan and purpose can be. Sometimes I think I understand it, but then other times I consider there must be more to it. I am certain that God is working—and somehow, some way, all this will be for His glory. But that doesn't make it any easier. One day during a walk, these reflections churned in my mind, and I started talking to God.

"Is this all there is, or is there another purpose?" I asked.

That same voice responded, *They're watching.*

I don't know who "they" are, but there is someone watching me. How I handle this battle will impact someone's life.

I believe that God's plan is perfect and unchanging. He has a singular plan, but that plan encompasses more than one purpose. Every day I continue this voyage, I turn another page in God's plan. His purpose may change from day to day, but I must be prepared and available every day to be a part of God's purpose.

UNCERTAINTY

June 3, 2012

There have been a few nights lately when I wake up and can't go back to sleep. I will toss and turn, and with each flip, another question comes to mind.

How long will this medicine work?

Will I live to be fifty-five or one hundred five?

How come the medicine has been so effective for me?

Will I know if the cancer comes back?

I realize these questions have one thing in common: uncertainty. I've always known my plans—where I'd go and what I would do. I don't function well with uncertainty, and now it seems like the only certainty is uncertainty. There are no answers for the questions that swirl through my mind.

At times, my life seems to be a storm of uncertainty. But in the storm, there is One I can turn to who is certain. He continues to walk with me and guide me through this mess. He's lifted me up and placed my feet on solid ground. He knows where I've been and where I'm going before I do. I'm thankful that Jesus is here to calm the storm.

What about you? Do you have anyone that you can turn to when the storms of life threaten to pull you under? If not, seek out Jesus.

LESSONS FROM A DEAD BATTERY

June 9, 2012

I've gotten bored riding my fixie around the neighborhood and decided it was time to venture out. This morning, the time felt right to hit the roads for a little ride. Since I hadn't ridden my road bike for several months, I had to reinflate the tires and find all my bike-riding stuff. I walked my bike down the sidewalk to the street and, as per my usual routine, I pressed the bike computer's start button to begin tracking my ride distance and speed. A blank screen stared back at me. Using my astute engineering mind, I pressed the button a second and third time, expecting a different response. Nothing. Finally, I realized the battery was dead and decided I'd just enjoy the ride and not worry about how fast and how far I was riding.

As I rode along, I instinctively glanced at the computer to check my progress. It finally hit me that although I knew my destination, I wouldn't know how far I had come, how far I had to go, or how fast I would get there. I'm still surprised when, where, and how God teaches me a lesson. Through that dead battery came a lesson about fighting cancer.

As I pedaled along, I realized this cancer fight isn't much different than living life. On the timeline of my life, I know my final destination but not how far I've come, how far I have to go, or how fast I'll get there.

Other than being confident of my final destination, that isn't much different than everyone else's situation. None of us know how long our journey on this earth will be. No one is promised tomorrow. All we can do is lock down our final destination.

I'm praying that you have the assurance of knowing your final destination.

NO SMELL OF FIRE

June 20, 2012

Several months ago, I read through the book of Daniel. I still enjoy reading the old Bible stories, but sometimes my familiarity with the stories causes me to overlook some of the lessons that God wants me to learn. I'm learning that whenever I miss the lesson, God will eventually lead me back.

This was the case with the story of Shadrach, Meshach, and Abednego. The story of their trial is told in Daniel 3. Shadrach, Meshach, and Abednego's refusal to acknowledge the king as a god and bow to his figure has led them to face their trial. The king has them bound and thrown into a fire that's so hot, the soldiers throwing them in died. However, when the king looks into the fire, he sees four men—not just the three who were thrown in. I personally believe that the fourth man was the Lord. What I get from this is that the Lord doesn't just lead us to our trials and then abandon us to flounder around on our own. He's in there with us through our trials. I also noticed the three men were bound by soldiers before being thrown into the fire; however, the king sees them walking around loose in the fire. Although they were tied up when thrown into the fire, that same fire burned off the bounds.

These past two years, I've been frustrated at times by the restrictions I now face, but now I realize God doesn't use our trials to bind us but to set us free from that which has us bound.

When the king tells the men to come out of the fire, all the high officials gather around. They notice the men have been protected from the fire and that no physical harm has come to them or their clothing. They also notice there isn't even the smell of fire.

And that's the way with my current trial. If you were to meet me on the street, you wouldn't be able to tell I have lung cancer. Just like Shadrach, Meshach, and Abednego, the only way you would know my story is for me to tell you. Here we are thousands of years later, and we still know the story of these men. Telling our story is the only way other people will know of our trials and God's actions on our behalf.

I also noticed that Shadrach, Meshach, and Abednego's lives were never the same. My Bible says the king caused them to prosper in the province of Babylon. Had they not gone through this trial, they wouldn't have received the blessings that came after.

There are times I'd like to have my life back to the way it was, but then I wonder what blessings I'd miss out on if I wasn't going through this trial. The telling of an old story has taught lessons leading to a new story to be told.

PRUNING

August 20, 2012

At our first house in Midland, Texas, we wanted rose bushes in the backyard. I bought a book that told how to properly feed, water, care for, and prune rose bushes. Then we planted six of them in the flower beds. As long as I paid attention to the bushes, they grew rapidly and produced beautiful roses well into the fall. However, problems occurred when I didn't keep up with the pruning. The branches grew out instead of up, and before long, other bushes became intertwined and entangled. Pruning became difficult. I had to begin with small cuts and then work my way into the bush. Once properly reshaped, the roses became tall and beautiful again.

I've started to realize that a life with Christ is a great deal like those rose bushes. There are times we can grow straight and beautiful. Then there are times we don't pay attention, and things in life begin to grow together and get all tangled up. The Master Gardener needs to come along and do some pruning. That pruning can hurt—a lot. After He's done cutting out the old tangled and ugly branches, we can, once again, begin to grow straight and beautiful.

There's been a lot of pruning the last two years. Just when I think it's all done, Jesus finds another branch that needs to be pruned. Initially, that snipping has been painful, but over time, it's become a relief to have the old cut away so the new can grow. I'm looking forward to being the rose bush that Jesus wants me to be.

DEEP ROOTS

August 29, 2012

I was spending another early Sunday morning in the living room, as I'd been awake for several hours, tossing and turning in bed before finally giving up. This was because just three days earlier, I had learned my work group was being disbanded and that I needed to find a new job. For hours, I was running the what-ifs through my head, trying to figure out where money could come from in the event I couldn't find another job. Just how many hits am I expected to take?

After eating breakfast, I turned on Dr. David Jeremiah to watch his message. Wouldn't you know it? It was about deepening our faith. I swear this man is following me. He told a story about two farmers who lived on separate sides of a mountain. This mountain was known for the bad storms that swept over it. Both farmers had decided to plant new crops of trees. The older farmer planted his and then pretty much left nature to take its course on them. The younger farmer on the other side of the mountain planted his trees and watered them regularly. He then carefully built berms around each tree to hold the water. He even told the older farmer that he should be taking better care of his trees. The older farmer just nodded and said they'd be okay. The younger farmer's trees grew and bloomed. The older farmer's trees looked like they were just getting by.

Then one night a storm hit. The rains poured, and the wind blew. The next morning, the younger farmer's trees were all down, their shallow roots exposed. The older farmer's trees were still standing. The younger farmer's trees had become dependent on the shallow water he had been delivering to them. The older farmer's trees had been forced to grow their roots deeper to find water, enabling them to withstand the storms. What had appeared to be indifference by the farmer had made them stronger and prepared for the storm he knew was coming.

In that one story, we can see two paths in the Christian life. There are those who believe and teach that once you become a Christian, all will be well. Jesus will come by and feed and water you. It will just be an easy life. Unfortunately, for those who think the road will be easy, they're toppled when the storm hits, and their roots are exposed. They've never grown the deep roots needed to survive such a storm.

The other path is that the Christian life isn't easy. It can be hard. It can contain pain and discomfort. Jesus has never promised the road would be easy. He only promised He'd be there with us. I think that Jesus uses the trials that enter our lives to encourage us to grow deeper roots. Jesus knows the storms that will enter our lives and uses each to make our roots go deeper to find the living water that only He can give.

I once thought that Jesus used the first fifty years of my life to prepare me to fight cancer. Perhaps, but now I believe He used these last two years of my life to deepen my roots to weather this latest storm. After witnessing all that Jesus has done these past two years, I believe He can also get me through this storm.

PICKING UP BREAD CRUMBS

January 6, 2013

During my last visit to MD Anderson, we learned my CT scan showed a suspicious spot on my right lung that's indicative of a new tumor. The doctors are uncertain if it's cancer and recommend a PET scan at my next appointment to reach a diagnosis. If the spot is cancer, that means it's found a way around the inhibitor drug I've been taking for the past twenty-two months.

From the beginning, we were informed there was no assurance of how long the medicine would work. I've done my best to push those thoughts out of my mind. Beating lung cancer once is hard enough. Beating it twice would be more difficult. When you're fighting cancer, you focus on the present and not what you may have to face tomorrow. However, now I have to begin thinking about what may lie ahead. Is there yet another bend in the road in this quest to beat the disease?

In seeking to look ahead, I find myself spending more time in the past. I keep replaying these last two and a half years. They've been nothing short of an incredible miracle. I've taken the medicine for twice as long as the average patient in any of the clinical trials. I've accomplished things that have the doctors shaking their heads and making statements like, "You're not typical."

As good as that may be, I still feel like I've missed something. I feel like maybe the disciples did in John 6. Jesus performed an incredible miracle by feeding over five thousand people with five loaves of bread and two small fish. Once everyone was fed and satisfied, Jesus told the disciples to go pick up the leftovers. He told them to let nothing go to waste. I don't think He was only talking about the food. I think Jesus wanted them to see with how much abundance He had met their needs.

As I've been reflecting on these past two and a half years and picking up the bread crumbs, there's one thing I'm seeing consistently: Jesus has been far ahead of us the whole time. He's known from the beginning what was to come and laid the stones for us to walk on. He knows what the results of the PET scan will be and is already preparing the path we will take.

MOUNTAINTOPS AND VALLEYS

January 12, 2013

I've learned on my quest to beat lung cancer, that in addition to bends in the roads, there are also mountaintops and valleys.

Mountaintops are the good days when I can see what I have and focus on that instead of what I need. Mountaintops are addictive. I fight like crazy to get to them. I fight even harder to stay there.

I've been able to enjoy more mountaintops than valleys these last two years. There's no way to go from mountaintop to mountaintop without passing through a valley. I've forgotten just how fast, rocky, and treacherous the descent into a valley can be. Now, here I am, again, in a valley. New spots are on my lung, and I'm in the hospital with pneumonia. Hitting the bottom hurt, and all I can see are shear, jagged cliffs. I don't see an easy path to begin climbing back to the mountaintop. I realize that, eventually, I'll get up, dust myself off, and start walking the road that's in front of me. I will either find the path back to the top, or I'll find the rich, lush part of the valley where the river flows to bring living water and nourishment to the valley. There, too, I'll be nourished and grow.

I'm beginning to believe that God doesn't intend for me to climb my way out of every valley. Sometimes the best way is to learn to grow my way out.

GRAPEFRUIT

January 27, 2013

I don't remember when I first began enjoying grapefruit for breakfast. I have an early childhood memory of seeing my dad eating it one Sunday morning. I tried a piece and liked it. From then on, for Sunday-morning breakfast, my dad and I would share a grapefruit. I continued to enjoy it at breakfast through adulthood.

Why the sudden memory of grapefruit? For the past twenty-two months, I haven't been allowed to eat it because of the cancer medicine. This is one of the weird things about grapefruit. For some reason, it can affect the way the medicine is metabolized in the body. The day after beginning the clinical trial drug, we went down to the breakfast buffet. There they were—grapefruit halves. I was really tempted, but I turned my back and haven't really thought about eating a grapefruit since—until last week.

When we learned the drug was no longer working, we started making preparations to begin a new clinical trial. I was taken off the cancer medicine to begin a washout period for seven to ten days before starting the new medicine. I decided I wanted grapefruit for breakfast. For the past few days, it's been restored to my life. I've already been told that when I begin the new medicine, it will, once again, be off the menu. I'll enjoy it while I can.

These past few days, I've regained a small part of my precancer life. Even though the cancer has returned, I still believe that, in time, God is going to restore the years the cancer has taken. Just like He restored the grapefruit.

ARMOR FITTING

February 9, 2013

We all know the story about David and Goliath. It's the story that inspires us to go out, overcome our fear to take on the big guy, and not avoid our biggest problems. However, there's a part of the story that gets skipped over that's helped me bring my fight against cancer into a new light.

Goliath has, once again, challenged the Israelites to send out their best warrior to fight him. David hears him and goes to King Saul's tent to tell the king he will fight Goliath. King Saul sees David standing there in his shepherding clothes and decides to give David his armor. Once the armor is placed on him, David tries to walk and realizes the armor isn't fitted for him. He's unable to even walk. David decides the best battle plan is to fight Goliath with his slingshot, five smooth stones, and his faith.

King Saul's armor would never have worked for David. If he had tried to use it, he would have failed.

I can see that God has uniquely fitted me with armor for my battle against cancer. The past few weeks, I've received multiple comments about my attitude and how I'm choosing to go through this battle. That's just the way I am, and I don't know any other way to do it. Trying to fight this cancer the way someone else has fought their cancer just cannot work for me. That would be like David trying to wear Saul's armor. I wouldn't be able to walk this road.

How many times have we heard inspirational stories from people and then gone out on the mission we think God has for us, only to fail? We can gain inspiration from other people, but we can't put on their faith or armor to fight our battles. Their armor isn't fitted for us. God knows the plans He has for us and the battles we will face. He will fit each of us for those battles with the armor He knows we'll need.

PUT ME IN, COACH

March 20, 2013

I love baseball. I've loved the game since I was six years old. Baseball was the first sport I was allowed to play. Back then, T-ball and coach pitch hadn't been invented, so we played baseball just like the big boys. Some of my earliest memories revolve around baseball. To this day, I can still remember my first real hit and how the ball shot off my bat into left field. I think the movie *The Sandlot* is loosely based on my childhood, because that was how we spent our summers. From sunup to sundown, we played baseball.

When Shane was home for spring break from college, we found time to play catch in the backyard. We haven't been able to play catch for a long time. I found I still love the feel of the glove on my hand, the way the laces of the ball feel as they roll off my fingertips, and how the ball feels as it pops the glove. I love the smell of the leather and the sound the ball makes when it lands squarely in the pocket of the glove. A game of catch brings back some good memories.

John Fogerty released the song "Centerfield" in 1985. This is one of the greatest baseball songs of all time. The lyrics remind me of my more youthful days, as it reflects how I approached every game. When I arrived, I was ready to play. My coaches never had to ask.

Fighting cancer is like the game of baseball. I have to get up every morning ready to play. There are no off days. I have to be ready even in the clinics and doctors' offices. I'm constantly meeting people suffering with and without cancer. I have to be ready to tell my story and the hope I have in Jesus. Maybe, just maybe, cancer is the way God has of putting me in the game.

Think how different life could be if we would love people more often who are suffering. We could make a difference if, every morning, we woke up and said, "Put me in, Coach. I'm ready to play today."

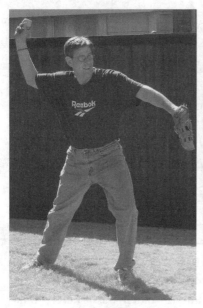 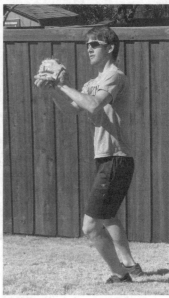

WHEN DREAMS INTERSECT

April 30, 2013

May of 2011 seems so far away right now, but that's when I first told you about Chad's dreams of racing bicycles professionally.

Chad raced much of 2011 on an elite amateur team out of Fort Collins, Colorado, and he had considerable success. The Kelley Benefits pro team liked what they were seeing and signed him for the remainder of the 2011 season. He rewarded them by finishing third overall in his first stage race with them. The team later rebranded to Optum Pro Cycling, and Chad signed with them for the 2012 season. His dream of being a professional cyclist was coming true.

Chad started 2012 with high expectations of himself. However, he returned from races in Uruguay and Guatemala sick and having to fight off illnesses that prevented him from racing. He also was involved in multiple crashes, and in a race in Canada, he injured his knee, which needed time to heal. He finally recovered from his illnesses and injuries and was getting into late-season form.

Then in July, he was entered in a stage race in Bend, Oregon. We received his call on Tuesday evening just after completing the prologue, which is a short time trial. He had won and would start the next day in the leader's yellow jersey—his first while on a pro team. Wednesday evening he called to inform us that he had been involved in another crash. His right thumb and left wrist were broken, and both would require surgery. He was deflated and heartbroken. His season was over.

The team made arrangements to have him flown back to Dallas on Thursday. We picked him up at the airport around midnight. His mother made an appointment with a hand specialist for early Friday morning. After a few hours' sleep, we were on the way to the doctor's office. The doctor confirmed surgery would be required to repair the injuries. By noon that same day, Chad was in surgery. They placed a screw in his left wrist and several pins in his right thumb. I was leaning on the bed rail when he started to wake up after surgery. He looked at me and said, "I was going to win that race."

The only words of wisdom I could offer were, "Sometimes, life just sucks."

It would be at least six weeks before Chad would be cleared to ride on the road again. He decided to stay with us to recuperate. Although he couldn't ride on the road, he could still ride on a trainer inside. With his time trial bike secured to a trainer, he rode with his elbows resting on the handle bars. I could tell he was working out his frustrations upstairs because the house would shake with the vibrations from the trainer.

Having to go through struggles myself was hard, but watching Chad having to go through his struggle was more difficult. I began to wonder if I had offered him good advice to pursue his dream and if his dream was coming to an end. Optum reassured Chad they wanted him back for 2013. Just a few weeks later, Chad was fitted with braces that would allow him to begin riding on the road again. But he would do no more road races in 2012. He returned to Colorado to resume his training and to start preparing for 2013.

During Chad's ordeal, I was still in the clinical trial for crizotinib. The drug had been highly effective at stopping my lung cancer. I'd been on the drug for twenty-two months, and I was beginning to dream of the day God would completely remove this disease from my life. Just before Christmas, my CT scan showed signs the cancer was returning, but the results were inconclusive. A PET scan and biopsy would be scheduled for my next appointment in January.

Both boys were home for Christmas, and we did our best to ignore the latest report.

In January, there I was, going through those blasted tests again. The PET scan showed increased cancer activity, but we had to wait on the biopsy pathology report to confirm cancer had returned. We discussed with the doctor other treatment options. DeLayne and I prayed that God would direct the path we should take by closing the door to options that weren't the right choice at this time and open the door to the trial He wanted me in.

The most promising drug was LDK378, but it had just completed the phase I trials and was closed. No one had the phase II trial open yet. There was another drug, HSP90, which was showing some promise. The closest place we were able to find it available was in a clinic in Fayetteville, Arkansas. My doctor referred me to the Highlands Oncology Group in Fayetteville.

That evening after the biopsy, I was, once again, sick and in the ER. I was admitted to the hospital for several days. We started for home Monday morning, and while we were stopped for lunch, I received a call from the clinic in Fayetteville. The clinical trial coordinator was touching base to give us her contact information in case the pathology report came back positive for cancer. I asked to confirm that this was for the HSP90 trial. She replied, "No, that trial just closed. This is for the LDK378 trial we just opened."

Tuesday morning we received the news that the pathology report showed cancer. Chad had just left for Colorado to try and beat the nasty winter storm about to hit Dallas. I found myself fighting back tears as I called the boys to tell them the battle was on again. Next I called the research assistant in Fayetteville and scheduled appointments for the following week. God was clearly opening the door to Fayetteville, but why, of all the clinics that were trying to open the trial in the United States, was this little clinic first?

I was accepted into the trial. Just two weeks later, I became the first patient in the United States to begin taking LDK378 as part of the phase II trial. The scans completed at my eight week follow-up showed the drug was working. The cancer activity was significantly reduced. My dream of beating cancer restored, we called the boys to tell them the good news. While talking to Chad, we told him my next appointment would be the week of April 22. He said that if we could hang around a couple of days after the appointment, he'd be in Fayetteville for the Joe Martin Stage Race. We decided to stay to watch him race since we hadn't seen him since January and had never seen him race in person with a pro team.

The year had started with a bang for Chad, who saw success in early races and finished second overall in a stage race in Portugal—his first European race. He returned from Portugal and then won the yellow leader's jersey in the individual time trial in the Redland's Classic in California. He held on to the yellow jersey until the final stage. He then had a couple of weeks to recover before heading for Arkansas.

The day after my doctor's appointment, we were in Devil's Den State Park to watch the first stage of the race. A short three-mile uphill time trial would take the pros just barely over eight minutes to finish. Chad found himself in second place—behind by just two seconds and ahead of third place by five seconds.

While stage one had been completed in almost perfect weather, stage two would be an incredible 110 miles in nasty, cold, drizzly, damp, and windy conditions. The group mainly stayed together, but once they hit downtown Fayetteville, Chad's team put in an amazing pull at the front to deliver their sprinter to the finish. Their acceleration was so sudden, it created a split in the field. Their effort fell just short with their sprinter finishing second. Unbeknownst to them, the yellow jersey race leader didn't make the split. Chad's team decided to ride back to the hotel, and we caught a ride back in the team van. On the way back to the hotel, phones started ringing. The team director was looking for Chad. He was now the race leader, and they needed him back downtown for the yellow jersey presentation.

Chad would start stage three, a 114-mile circuit race, in the yellow jersey—his second of the season. It was once again going to be horrible, cold, damp, and very foggy weather to race in. Since it was a circuit race, the team director worked out a plan for DeLayne and me to get a lap each in the team car. It was a blast. It really was one of the most fun things I've done in a while. To see what these athletes put themselves through and to see the team working together was amazing. Chad's team did their job protecting him. He played it cool, waiting for the rider in second place to make his move. When he made his move, Chad was still strong enough to go with him. They finished the day with the same time. The team had successfully defended the yellow jersey. Chad would start the final stage in yellow.

Stage four would be a "crit" in downtown Fayetteville. (A criterium consists of several laps around a closed circuit.) Sunday was a bright, sunny day. The weather was the complete opposite from the last two days. Chad would start the day with just a five-second lead ahead of Francisco Mancebo, who was still in second place overall—the rider who had beaten him out of the yellow jersey on the final day just a couple of weeks earlier.

The Optum guys started the stage out strong, controlling the front of the main group and keeping Chad out of trouble. A small group of riders was allowed to get a break that went out to forty-five seconds at one point, but Chad's teammates kept them in sight and slowly began to bring them back. With just two laps to go, the break was down to fifteen seconds. Chad was still close to the front. On the final lap, the group was all together with Mancebo ahead of him. It was up to Chad to not let a gap form between him and Mancebo. Chad and his team did their jobs and successfully defended the yellow jersey. Chad had just won the Joe Martin Stage race—his first National Racing Calendar win.

After seeing Chad cross the finish line, I let out a big yell, saw his team director, and gave him a hug. I then started toward the team van, where I knew Chad would be. Chad caught up to me about halfway there. He gave me a big hug and said, "That was for you. I love you and am so glad you're here to see it."

Then I knew that there, in downtown Fayetteville, God had allowed our dreams to intersect. Chad is a pro cyclist, and—if even for just that moment—I was healed of cancer.

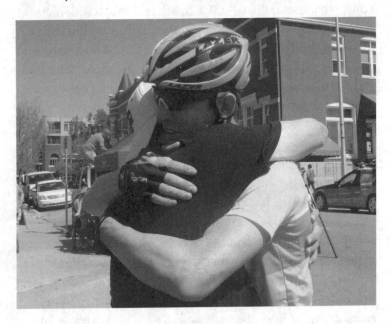

GOD AND PICKUP TRUCKS

July 14, 2013

It's now been three years ago this month that my journey to beat lung cancer began. In this time, I've learned a lot about God, Jesus, and myself. When I look back, I can clearly see where God has opened and closed doors as necessary and carried me when I needed it most. He has truly been involved in the biggest moments of my battle. But what about the small areas of my life? Does God really care about what I drive to work each day?

My Avalanche was ten years old, and it had been a good truck. However, I was beginning to have the feeling I was rolling on borrowed time. The value had dropped low enough that if I had to have it repaired, the cost could easily be 25 percent of the value of the truck. I'd never get that money back. I also thought it would be good to have another vehicle to drive to Fayetteville and stop racking up the miles on DeLayne's car. Since I wasn't in a rush to buy anything, I decided it was time to start looking. I began my research by visiting dealer web pages to see what used trucks were available and at what price.

I found a 2012 truck on a dealer's lot in Frisco and decided to stop after church on Sunday to check it out. They had two trucks that would fit my needs, so I scheduled test drives for Wednesday evening. When we arrived, we learned that the guy we were to see was on vacation, and that one of the trucks had been sent for recall repair work. Things went downhill from there. This dealership did nothing to improve the image of the stereotypical used-car salesman.

After we left, we stopped by another lot just to see what they had. They had one truck that matched my criteria, and we drove it. I wasn't ready to buy that night and had other trucks I wanted to look at. When we got home, I was feeling I should just stick with my old truck. I asked God to direct our decision.

The next day, I looked at more web pages of dealers down in Richardson and along I-75 in Dallas. I found one truck worth looking at, so we drove to the dealership. We noticed some damage on the truck, and I quickly lost interest.

We then headed toward Dallas to look in other car lots. As we approached one dealership, I told DeLayne, "I forgot about these guys." I saw two Chevy trucks on the lot, so we pulled in and were met by a salesman. When we reached the trucks, he showed us a 2013 model with just 5,500 miles on it. We liked it and asked if we could take it for a drive. While he went to get the keys, DeLayne and I discussed the deal we would try to get and what we wanted the bottom-line number to be. After the test drive, I asked the salesman to work up a deal for us to look at, still saying I wasn't sure I was ready to buy. He took the keys to my truck for them to do an appraisal.

Oh boy, now the fun begins, I thought.

After about fifteen minutes, he returned with a completed deal sheet and went through it. When he told us the bottom line number, I about fell out of the chair. Their initial offer was within $57 of where we wanted to be.

"What do you think about that?" he asked.

I wanted to say, "Sold!" but responded with, "You're really close to where I want to be."

I quickly decided to see what would happen if I were to use one of the old car-sales tactics on them. I shaved $557 off of their number and told him I would buy the truck that day if they hit that number, including tax, title, and license. He walked away and came back in five minutes.

"Chris, you just bought a truck."

As it turns out, the truck I bought was only two months old. The original owner had bit off more than he could chew on the payments and traded it for a less expensive car. The truck is much nicer than the first truck we had looked at, and the final deal was much better than we expected. It was less than the quote we had been given for two 2011 trucks with almost 26,000 miles on them!

I've stopped believing in coincidence a long time ago and believe that God was just as involved in this as He is in my fight against cancer. I believe it so much that I've nicknamed my new truck "The Miracle Truck."

God cares about every detail of our lives and wants better for us than we can imagine—even when it comes to what we drive to work.

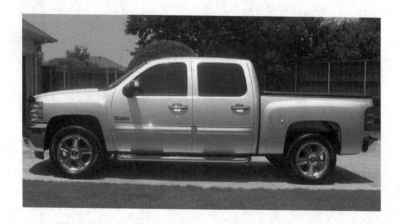

NO EVIDENCE OF DISEASE

September 29, 2013

I started taking LDK378 in mid-January, and eight months later, my scans, again, show no evidence of disease. For the second time in three years, with the help of the doctors, nurses, radiologists, medicine, and the grace of God, we've been able to defeat the beast in my chest. No one can anymore explain why I've had such a good response to the medicines as they can explain why I have lung cancer in the first place. I'm just one of those people—I'm not typical. It's given me much to think about.

For the past three years, I've seen a doctor every three to four weeks with scans every six to eight weeks. One thing I've noticed about fighting cancer: There's a lot of idle time in the waiting room and during tests. I spend my idle time thinking. I want and seek so desperately to find the answers and to understand the reasons we're traveling the road we're on. But I don't have any more of the answers than I did three years ago.

I think about the countless people we've met on this road who needed to be encouraged. Had it not been for my journey, I wouldn't have been able to encourage them. Often, the people who need some encouragement are the people who have come to treat me. The thought came to me that these people deal with and see so much death, they also need to see life.

I believe God is trying to teach me something through this experience. As I sit and think about these past three years, I'm beginning to wonder, *Did God allow cancer to enter my body so He could more fully teach me the depths of His love for me?* That's a real mind-bender. Does God allow trials to enter our lives in order to bless us and others through those trials?

All I know is, if I didn't have cancer, I would've missed so many blessings. Without cancer, I wouldn't see God the way I see Him today.

Long before I had cancer, I had another deadly disease—sin. As I've contemplated beating cancer a second time, I'm struck by the parallel between my physical battle and my spiritual condition. Physically, when the doctors look at me, they see no evidence of disease. Spiritually, when God looks at me, He sees no evidence of the disease of sin—only because of the saving grace provided by Jesus' death on the cross.

TOUGH AS LEATHER

December 3, 2013

When I was in middle school, I took my first shop class. One of the things we were taught was how to tool leather. We learned how to take leather pieces, put designs in them, and stitch them together. I really enjoyed making things and continued to do so through high school and even into college. I made wallets and belts for family and friends. I was good enough at it that the owner of a local western store offered me an opportunity to sell belts in his store. I knew how long it took to make a good one and didn't see where I could make enough to make any money at it. Besides, when you start selling your hobby, it becomes work.

I put the tools away after college, and they've since been stored in a closet in every house we've lived in. When Shane was in middle school, he wanted to know how to tool leather. I had some scrap pieces of leather stored with the tools, and we broke them out. I started teaching him how to cut and stamp the leather. Also stored with the tools was a wallet kit. I started tooling it but didn't finish it up. Eventually, we put it all back in the closet.

This year, I decided to take all of Thanksgiving week off as vacation. Then I saw the weather forecast was for cold, damp, and rainy weather, and I had planned to do things outside. What was I going to do? The unfinished wallet came to mind. I decided to get it and my tools out again. When I saw the leather back of the wallet, I could tell it was dried out. It had been close to ten years since I started that wallet. It would need to be prepared properly before I would be able to tool it. In leather-work, preparing a piece of leather for working is called casing. The way I learned to do it was by using a sponge to apply water to the leather to get it damp and then sealing the leather in a plastic bag. This lets the pores of the leather open up. Then the leather will get soft. Without casing, the tools wouldn't leave their imprints in the leather, and it would be difficult to work with. Once the leather was cased, I was able to finish cutting and stamping the leather. I'm not as good at it as I used to be, but the wallet is almost finished and ready for stitching.

As Christians, I think that sometimes we believe we're as tough as that dry piece of leather. God can't work with us like that, and we won't accept his imprint on our lives. We need to be cased before he can really work with us. That's where our trials come in. We tend to think that God has forsaken us.

Often, hard times aren't the absence of God but evidence of His presence in our life. It's during these times that God is preparing us to receive His imprint.

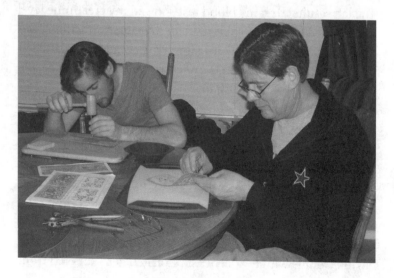

THE BEST

March 30, 2014

Have you ever had a period in your life where it seemed like everything you prayed about seemed to be getting worse? Well, that's where I've been for several weeks. I was physically exhausted and mentally frustrated from trying to keep all the balls in the air. The question formed in my mind, *Just how long can I keep all this up?* I was praying that somewhere, somehow, God would give me a break from something. Little did I know what I was asking for.

I'd just been to Fayetteville on Monday and left thinking that everything was going just fine medically. Thursday afternoon, I received an unexpected call from the clinical trial coordinator. The lab results from my blood test showed my creatinine level had reached an unacceptable level for my kidney function. I was told to stop taking the trial drug immediately and get retested in five days. Then, based upon the retest results, they would decide how to proceed with treatment.

God, this isn't the break I was looking for.

A few months ago, I was looking for any new information on LDK378 and came across a blog by a young mother who had just started the drug. Earlier this week, I decided to check her blog to see how she was doing and found she was still struggling with the side effects. I sent her an email describing the ways I had found most effective in getting through the day. She responded with a thank-you email and also mentioned she was having trouble with headaches. I informed her I suffered from those too. She's the only other LDK378 patient I've communicated with. Since we had similar side effects, I asked her if she had seen a change in her creatinine levels.

She responded to my question and then gave me some unexpected advice: "Enjoy your time off the medicine and use it as a time to rest and physically recover."

She was right.

After reading her advice, I realized that for the first time in four years, I'm not taking medicine to fight cancer or the side effects of those drugs. I'm not taking medications for pain, pneumonia, nausea, intestinal issues, or blood clots. I also don't have cancer! I've been able to go through the days not ruled by the medicine and watching the clock to see when I could eat. I've been able to sleep in later this weekend instead of waking up early to keep on my medication schedule. We've been able to go out and enjoy a movie and dinner without taking pills in my pocket. It's amazing that in just four short years, I've forgotten what life without cancer is like.

While enjoying this break, I've also been reminded that when I began taking this medicine, we knew it was probably not something I'd be able to take long term. Like with crizotinib, there would come a time when it would begin to fail or cause toxicity problems. I also knew that, just like the crizotinib, God wouldn't allow it to fail until a better medicine was available. Have we now reached that point, or is this just a little bump in the road? I don't know, but I do know that God wants the best for me.

If His best is for me to continue this medicine, even on a reduced dose, then that will happen. If His best is for me not to continue on this medicine, then we will continue on this path, knowing His best lies on whatever road He directs us. I also know that when the time comes that His best is no longer available on this earth, then—and only then—will my journey end. I will go home to receive His very best.

LEARNING TO FLY

April 6, 2014

Last summer, I was looking out our kitchen window and had the chance to watch a momma bird teaching her baby bird to fly. They were perched on the fence together when Momma bird took off, flew out and back, and then landed on the fence about five feet from the baby. The baby bird looked at its momma and hopped down the fence line, stopping next to Momma. The process had repeated at least three times when Momma bird took off and flew to a tree about five feet away. The baby bird just sat on the fence and chirped. I found myself rooting for the baby bird. "Come on, you can do it—fly."

The baby finally stretched its wings and flapped a couple of times and then flew over to the momma. That little five-foot flight had just opened a new world to that baby bird. I'm sure it wasn't much longer until the baby bird was out of the nest.

As I think about that scene playing out, I realize it's not much different for us as parents. From the time our children are born, we protect them and take steps to prepare them to leave our nest and fly out into the world on their own. We often use terms like "leave the nest" or "empty nesters" to describe the process. There are times that we doubt ourselves and wonder if our kids are ever going to get it. Why are they content to just hop when they have the ability to fly? Then one day, they spread those wings and are gone, and you believe they're set on a trajectory for their life.

Sometimes they make a decision you didn't see coming.

That's what we've experienced with Shane the past few weeks. For several years now, we thought Shane would follow his brother into the pro bike racing circuit. He had already taken the first step by signing a contract with a domestic professional team. However, after a few months, Shane decided that pro racing wasn't for him. I'll admit being a little surprised at his decision. But since being diagnosed with cancer, I've told the boys to find something they really enjoy doing so they will look forward to going to work. I was impressed at how he sought wise counsel from his friends and family. He also prayed and asked God for His guidance. He's spreading those wings on his own.

I realized that DeLayne and I invested twelve years in Shane-the-baseball-player, five years in Shane-the-cyclist, but we've invested twenty-three years in Shane, the man. Shane and I spent a lot of time together during those years, and I was given an opportunity not afforded to many fathers. I was able to watch my son grow from a boy into a young man.

Just after the first of the year, Shane talked me into going out for a short bike ride with him. As we rode, I noticed he positioned himself to block me from the wind. I realized we had crossed a threshold into a new chapter in life due to cancer. The protector had become the protected.

NOT LETTING GO

June 16, 2014

My symptoms first began to appear over four years ago. I didn't know or understand much about the journey that I was beginning to take—where it would go or how long it would last. I'm amazed at how my memories of events from years ago have been used to teach me lessons along this road.

These past few weeks, a memory has kept popping into my head. The memory is from the days that Chad had his learner's permit, and we were teaching him how to drive. At the time, I was driving the truck that was destined to be his when he turned sixteen. In fact, he even helped pick out the truck when we bought it. One Saturday morning, I awoke early and looked out the window to see the grass and streets covered with snow. I thought this would be a great opportunity to teach Chad to drive on icy streets. In North Texas, snow doesn't last long, so I went out and cleaned off the truck. Then I went up to Chad's room and rousted him out of bed. "Get up, we're going driving."

At the time, there was a new neighborhood going in across the street from our neighborhood. All the streets were in, but no houses were built yet. I drove across to that neighborhood. Then we switched places. I had Chad drive around the streets. Every now and then I'd tell him to give it a little extra gas around the corner so the back end would slide out, and he'd have to correct the slide. Once I felt like he had a good grasp of how to drive in these conditions, I had him drive down to the end of the longest

154

street in the neighborhood and turn around. He was centered in the middle of the street.

"I want you to speed up to thirty miles per hour and then slam on the brakes," I said.

Chad looked at me with a look of concern. What I had just told him to do was a complete contradiction to what I'd been telling him for almost thirty minutes. Not to mention, it sounded like I wanted him to turn his future truck into a sled.

I repeated my instructions, but this time I added, "No matter what you feel, don't let go."

I knew what was about to happen, but Chad hadn't experienced anti-lock brakes before. He did as I instructed, and things went just as I knew they would. Driving lesson complete, we headed for home.

Now, what does that story have to do with cancer? Of late, there've been several occasions when I start to lose my focus. There doesn't seem to be anything positive. When all I see is impending chaos, I feel like things are sliding out of control.

At those times, I can hear God say, *I've brought you to this place and put you on this journey for a reason. All you need to do is keep going. No matter what you feel, don't let go of Me.*

THIRTY YEARS

July 7, 2014

Thirty years ago, I stood at the front of a church and looked down the center aisle to see the love of my life slowly walking toward me. We had stuck with tradition. This was the first time I had seen her that day and the first time I'd seen her in her wedding gown. On that day, we promised we would love, honor, and cherish each other for richer, for poorer, in sickness, and in health.

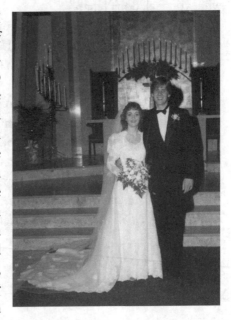

In the last thirty years, we've pretty well covered those bases.

We'd only been married two months when DeLayne was laid off from her job. There we were with my tuition bills to pay—and half our income was gone. That didn't last long, because DeLayne's very talented as a Certified Professional Secretary, and she was able to find another job quickly. At the time, I still had two more semesters left in college. Because of the money we were able to build up in our savings, I was able to quit my job and take all my remaining classes in that last semester. I had an engineering job offer locked down before graduation, and we were on our way.

Just one month after graduation, we packed everything up and moved to Midland, Texas, for my first real job. We joke now about how that was one of the decisions that made our marriage stronger. Moving twelve hours from our families meant we had only ourselves to depend on. Since we left all of our friends and family behind, it forced us two introverts to meet new people and make new friends. The friends that we made during those years are ones we still stay in touch with. Five years and one baby later, we packed up and moved again.

We made our second home in Sherman, Texas. Just seven months after moving, baby number two arrived. DeLayne delivered Shane just like she had Chad—no painkillers. At the hospital, I heard the best description ever of DeLayne. I came out of her room and bumped into the doctor who had just delivered Shane. As we walked to the nursery, he looked at me and said, "That DeLayne is as tough as an old worn boot."

The years we spent in Sherman were good years with my being promoted and earning an MBA. With that extra security, we decided the time was right for DeLayne to leave her job and start her own secretarial business based out of our home. Having her own business allowed DeLayne to keep her own schedule and be there when the boys got out of school. My job was going well, and I was soon offered a job in Dallas. We packed everything up and moved closer to Dallas.

My new job required that I travel to Asia twice a year. DeLayne was busy starting her business in McKinney but was still able to take up the slack created when one parent was missing. A few years after moving, DeLayne began having a minor medical problem. After being sent from one specialist to another with no diagnosis, one doctor ordered a CT scan. The report came back that there were spots in her liver. We were finally referred to a liver specialist in Dallas. I remember sitting in the waiting room, looking at people who were obviously ill and wondering, *Is this what our future looks like? And if it is, how am I going to be able to handle it?* When we saw the doctor, he just looked at DeLayne and said, "You have cysts in your liver. No big deal—lots of people have them. Go enjoy your life." Relieved, we left the doctor's office.

Little did we know, we had just seen a glimpse of our future.

From there, life went on. Both boys were busy in school and sports. DeLayne's business was going well, and my work and coaching the boys kept me busy. Before we knew it, Chad and Shane had graduated high school and were in college. Just like that, DeLayne and I had been married twenty-five years. Our lives were going just the way they were supposed to. We were looking forward to spending time together and to eventually retiring.

And then I began to cough. We started spending more time together, but not the way we had planned.

The first twenty-five years were preparation for what was to come. I knew life had just taken a drastic turn, and I wasn't sure how I was going to deal with it. Actually, I ended up with the easier part. DeLayne deserves better than the deal she's gotten. Being the caregiver to a cancer patient is much harder than being the cancer patient. All I have to do is lie there and be sick. DeLayne deals with keeping the schedule straight, handling the never-ending insurance paperwork, and maintaining my medical records. On top of that, she has to witness this mess.

One thing most people don't know is that it's very easy for a cancer patient to become overwhelmed. There are days when I just want to shut down. Situations that wouldn't have been a big deal before I got sick can frustrate the bejeebers out of me now. I can usually do a good job keeping it together around other people, but DeLayne lives with me and sees the ugly side of what cancer has done to me. She's there when I've had enough and the lid blows off in frustration, and she'll give me a needed hug.

I'm so thankful she's keeping the vow she made to me thirty years ago and that she's as tough as an old worn boot.

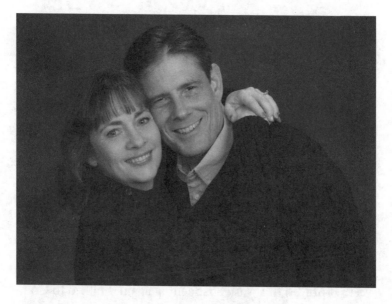

UNKNOWN LAND

August 27, 2014

The past twenty months have been pretty uneventful health-wise. There've been no trips to the emergency room and no hospital stays. Once we figured out my high fevers were caused by a reaction to the CT contrast, we've just been sailing along. The medical team in Fayetteville had become special friends to us, and we'd become comfortable with life on the smooth path.

And then I began to cough.

Four weeks ago, that familiar dry cough reappeared. Instinctively, I knew my medicine had started to fail. For the next three weeks, I prayed this wasn't happening again. I talked to God, telling Him that having to do this a third time could be more than I was prepared for.

"If it's Your will, don't let it be so," I prayed.

The CT scan conducted just a week ago confirmed there's a new area of concern in my right lung. The time has come to get back in the fight. It's time to move from the terrain we've become comfortable with. Unlike the last two times where the treatment path was clearly laid out in front of us this, this time we're staring down a path to the unknown. There are no drugs with solid test results for me to change to. Trying to decide on a treatment based on the results of one or two patients is a scary position to be in, but that's what we will have to do.

The Sunday morning we were packing for our last trip to Fayetteville, the words God spoke to Abram popped into my head. God told Abram to pack all his belongings and move to a "land that I will show you." Those words have been stuck in my head as we've been evaluating the different drug trials that are available. We've been seeking God's direction to find the best plan for me. While we've narrowed down the choices to two or three drugs, there still doesn't appear to be a clear path. We're heading into unknown land.

The one thing we do know is that God will show us the land we're to go to, and He will be waiting for us when we arrive.

A COLLECTION OF RANDOMNESS

September 30, 2014

It's been a little over four weeks now since I started in a phase I trial for X-396. I had a bad reaction to the medicine. My face was engulfed with a hot rash, and I seemed to be in never-ending extreme pain. The thought occurred to me this might be what hell is like—constant burning torment and no relief. Add eternal separation from God, and I think you'd be there. I'm thankful I know who my Savior is.

Due to the reaction, I was taken off of the drug for ten days to clear up the rash. The last two weeks have been very trying for me, as I haven't been able to make any sense of it all. I've wanted to write a new blog but haven't been able to put my thoughts together. So today I offer you my thoughts on some seemingly random events over the past few weeks.

While I was dealing with the rash, I had a lot of sleepless nights. One of those nights, I turned on the TV and started flipping channels. I happened across a minister who is very popular right now. I will only say that most of his teaching is based on the "name it, claim it" theology. As I listened to him, I began to feel sympathy for the people in his congregation who are fighting long-term health issues like I am. If I were to believe what he's teaching, the reason I haven't been healed from cancer is because I don't have enough faith.

Hogwash! I would suggest this minister read this:

> But as for me, my prayer is to You, O Lord, at an accept-
> able time; O God, in the greatness of Your lovingkindness,
> answer me with Your saving truth. Deliver me from the
> mire and do not let me sink; may I be delivered from my
> foes and from the deep waters.
>
> —PSALM 69:13–14

God doesn't operate on man's clock. At an acceptable time to God, He will answer our prayers out of His lovingkindness. Sometimes He says yes, sometimes no, and sometimes wait. Faith is knowing God will answer us out of His will.

—∿∿—

I was reading a commentary on hope the other day. Hope has gotten a bad rap lately. There are a lot of people who have placed their hope in a man. That man has now disappointed them in one way or another, and they've lost their hope.

The last few weeks, there have been days when hope is what has gotten me through the day. There have been days that hope is the only rope I have to hold on to. That rope has been frayed. At times, it feels like it's down to the last thread. The thing that keeps me going is knowing the other end of that rope is held by the nail-pierced hand of Jesus.

—∿∿—

One Sunday morning, I was watching a very well-known minister talking about encountering troubles in our lives. He was making the point that, as Christians, nothing comes to us that hasn't passed through God's hands. I believe that to be true, as well. However, there are times I wish God would hold His hands a little tighter together.

It had been another long day at MD Anderson Cancer Center. There had been a mix-up with my schedule and, once again, I was going to be delayed in taking the new trial drug. I'm not allowed to eat for two hours before taking the medicine. I hadn't eaten since early that morning. The longer things stretched on, the hungrier I got and the more my frustration built. Finally around two o'clock that afternoon, I was allowed to take the drug and leave the clinic. I'd had enough for one day and practically ran back to the truck. I wanted out of MDA and out of Houston as quick as I could.

I'm also not allowed to eat for two hours after taking the medicine. As we headed north on I-45 in stop-and-go traffic, the minutes just ticked by. We hit Huntsville just as it was time to eat. I needed some food, and the snacks in the truck wouldn't do. I wanted pancakes and found the local IHOP.

After our waiter brought us some water and took our order, I could feel the last bit of energy draining from my body as we sat in the booth. I put my head in the palms of my hands and closed my eyes for a few minutes. My momentary rest was interrupted by our waiter asking if I would like some orange juice for a little pick-me-up. "No charge." He had noticed the bandage on my arm and thought I'd just donated blood.

"No thanks on the orange juice," I told him, "but if you could find an orange, I'd really appreciate it."

I thought I had just asked the impossible. "No way he brings back an orange," I told DeLayne.

Just a few minutes later, here he came with a bowl of canned oranges. He apologized for them being canned. "We just got these in for some reason," he explained. They don't normally carry them.

DeLayne and I teared up a little. It wasn't about the oranges. It was that someone saw we weren't having a good day and took a few moments to care. Sometimes you may see someone in need and think that what you have to offer won't make a difference and move on. That small gesture may not mean much to you, but it may be the high point of that person's day.

CUPS

November 3, 2014

Last week we learned my treatment with X-396 wasn't working. I was removed from the clinical trial. As we were driving
home from Houston, my thoughts turned to . . . cups.

We have paper cups, plastic cups, and Styrofoam cups. There
are tea cups and coffee cups. You can have a cup of joe or a cup
of tea. Ever had a cup made of cake? Or what about a choco-
late peanut butter cup? Sometimes our cups are half full or half
empty. Has your cup ever overflowed?

For most of my life, I've been blessed with an overflowing
cup. I can't think of a time that my needs have never been met.
My cup has overflowed with friends and loved ones. I've been
blessed beyond measure so many times I can't count them all.

Four years ago, I was handed a different cup. This cup is not
of my choosing. There have been times this cup has been filled
with discomfort and pain. But then there are times it's been filled
with laughter and joy.

Recently, my cup has been filled with frustration, doubt, and
uncertainty. I pray every night for God to take this cup back. I
just can't drink any more from it. So far, He hasn't chosen to take
this cup from me. He tells me to look at my cup again.

There I see it. It's a little battered and bruised, but I still see
in my cup . . . hope.

UNBELIEF

November 16, 2014

A few months ago, I began to feel the lung cancer was returning again. I sensed this time it would be a real fight. Now, after having failed my third ALK inhibitor in just eight weeks, I can see that feeling was well-founded. Not only have I been experiencing more of a physical battle this time, but I've been experiencing a real challenge spiritually.

These past three weeks, I've had family and friends encouraging me to keep my faith and hope in Jesus. The thing is, as I reflect on what I believe now versus four years ago, I still believe the same things. I believe that God, at a time of His choosing, can heal me. I believe by the stripes on Jesus' back that I've been healed. I stand strong on those pillars of faith. Still, I've noticed there's a struggle within me.

I've learned at times like these, it's best to just be quiet and listen. As I sat and listened, I heard one word: *unbelief.* As I thought about that word, I remembered a story in the Bible of a father who also needed help with his unbelief. The story is found in Mark 9:14–29. A father took his son to the disciples to be healed of a demon spirit. The disciples were unable to heal the boy. Then Jesus showed up. Jesus questioned the father about how long the boy had been like this.

And he said, "From childhood. It has often thrown him both into the fire and into the water to destroy him. But if You can do anything, take pity on us and help us!" And Jesus said to him, "'If You can?' All things are possible to him who believes." Immediately the boy's father cried out and said, "I do believe; help my unbelief!"

—MARK 9:21–24

What I believe has long since been settled. What I struggle with now are areas of my unbelief. The question is not, *Can God heal me?* or even, *Will God heal me?* The question is, *Where will God heal me?* Up until the past few weeks, I've believed God would heal me here on earth. But with the repeated diagnosis, there's now some doubt in that belief. My prayer is that Jesus shows up, takes pity on me, and helps me overcome my unbelief.

LIVING PSALM 13

May 17, 2015

Is there a scripture you find yourself continually being drawn back to? I've been on this journey to beat lung cancer for almost five years now. There have been more ups and downs than I can count. I've been in another clinical trial since November and currently have no evidence of disease for the third time. But the longer this battle has gone on, the more wary and frayed I've become. During this time, a scripture has emerged which I find myself relating to more and more frequently. I find myself reading it often. The scripture that's becoming dear to me is Psalm 13.

Psalm 13 was written by David. Each time I read it, I find myself thinking, *Wow, this is my life right now.* At the time David wrote this psalm, he was the anointed future king of Israel. Yet, there he was running for his life from King Saul, who sought to take his life. David, a man after God's own heart, was seeking refuge wherever he could find it. He was spending days and nights in dark and damp caves, never knowing when King Saul and his men would come. David was tired, exhausted, and he was seeking some answers. I can imagine David sitting alone at the top of a hill, feeling isolated from God, when he began to pour out his heart to God with the questions he'd been wrestling with.

Most of David's questions can be summed up with, "How long, O LORD, will this continue?" David already knew his future. He would one day be the king of Israel, but he was so tired of running, he just had to ask. David asked God the questions that had been weighing heavy on his heart.

The one thing that sticks out in this psalm is what's missing. Nowhere do I find that God answered any of David's questions. He didn't have to. In the final verse, David realized what God had already done for him. I can see David in a moment recalling the memory of his battle with Goliath and how with a single stone the giant was slain. He remembers how many times God has blessed him and rejoices.

The reason I can relate to this psalm is that cancer has become my King Saul. It seeks to take my life. Even though I've now beaten cancer three times, I never know when it will show up again. At night when I can't sleep, I find myself questioning God.

How long will this go on?

Why haven't you just healed me?

Sometimes I feel like I shouldn't question God's plan or will, but I don't think He's surprised by these questions. After all, if a man after God's own heart can ask these questions, why can't I? I don't get any answers either, because He doesn't need to answer.

Each time that cancer has shown its hideous face, God has provided a stone to slay the giant. I have to remind myself that God has continually laid the stones that have made the path I travel. I don't know how long this journey will last or where it will take me next. All I can do is pray that with each step I take, God has already placed the rock for me to step on.

VACATION!

July 18, 2015

After having been in practically nonstop treatment for almost five years and developing anxiety about my current treatment, my oncologist strongly suggested I take a break from chemo. We decided that after my last treatment in June, we would take the regularly scheduled week off. The following week we'd take a vacation to celebrate our thirty-first anniversary and five years of surviving lung cancer. I had my regularly scheduled scans, and then the next day we were off. It was nice to get a break from cancer and treatments, if only for a week.

We decided to fly up to Wyoming and visit Yellowstone National Park and Grand Teton National Park. We had a great time, and it gave me a chance to play with my camera again. Vacation came to an end way too soon, but it was good to get out and see some of God's handiwork.

While there, I couldn't help but think that the God who created all of this also created me. He knows the number of hairs on my head and the number of my days.

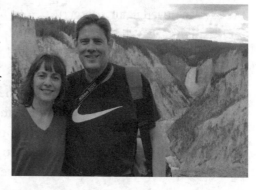

Most of all, He loves me.

MADE IT TO FIVE YEARS

August 31, 2015

On July 30 at 3:30 in the afternoon, it became official. Five years ago on that date and time is when I heard the words, "The pathology report confirms lung cancer." That evening, I thought, *Well, okay, I'll take this on as hard as I can and beat it. Then I'll go on and enjoy the rest of my life.*

I was terribly naive.

A few weeks later, I sat in an exam room to get the results of all the tests done the previous week. The cancer had already spread throughout my chest, and there was a brain tumor. The disease was stage IV. With those words, thirty-five more years of life expectancy were swept away. I had a 50 percent chance of living possibly one more year and a 1 to 4 percent chance of living another five years. However long I live, barring a miracle, I'll be in some kind of treatment. Having now made it five years, I've made it into that top 1 to 4 percent—the highest ranking I've ever achieved in anything.

The night I was diagnosed, I knelt in prayer and asked for three things. Now after five years, I thought it might be a useful exercise, mostly for myself, to revisit those three prayer requests and see how God has chosen to answer them.

The first thing I prayed for was for healing. We've now beaten back lung cancer three times. Only by God answering many, many prayers is that possible. Some people would consider that this request has been answered. However, in my own way,

I don't consider myself healed. I believe when I'm healed, I will no longer need to take drugs, and my collapsed lung will be restored.

I've really been drawn to the story of the man with the withered hand told in Matthew 12. In that story, Jesus tells the man with the withered hand to stretch out his hand, and, in an instant, the man's hand is completely healed. Even after five years, I still believe that it will be the same with me. In an instant, when Jesus says the words, my lung will be healed. But after five years, I have to admit that I now have to consider it may not be part of God's will to completely heal me. Even though that may be the case, I still go to bed each evening persistent in my prayer for complete healing. The longer the wait, the bigger the miracle will be.

The next thing I prayed for was that God would place the right people in the right place at the right time to help us fight lung cancer. Looking back through the years, I can plainly see how God has answered this prayer and still does. From people at the Cancer Encouragement Group we attend, to the doctors and medical staff who have treated me, God has placed each of these people there to help us. We've even had people at the hotel breakfast buffet pray for us, once they knew our story. I can't leave out the friends and family who have stepped in when we needed them. There have been many times these people have sat and listened to me whine about how I feel. I try not to add my problems to other people's problems, but I always feel better after I've had a chance to unload a little. There have been too many "right people" to list them all, but they are all very special to DeLayne and me.

The last thing I prayed for was that this cancer wouldn't go to waste. This is why I still consent to clinical trials and extra tests. Some of them have been painful and unpleasant experiences. Being first to find out the side effects isn't fun, but I want the doctors and pharmaceutical companies to learn as much as they can from me. It's worth it to meet someone who is experiencing good results from a drug or treatment that I was one of the first to test.

I've learned a lot in five years, but there are still some things I'm trying to figure out. I've heard several ministers say we should never ask God, "Why the trial?" He won't answer that question. But He will answer the questions about the purpose of trials. I'll admit, this is something I wrestle with almost daily. If God has answered the question of what the purpose of this trial is in our lives, either I haven't heard, or I'm as dumb as a box of rusty old hammers. I'm still just not getting it. It's possible I never will.

It's quite possible I won't understand all this until I open my eyes and see Jesus.

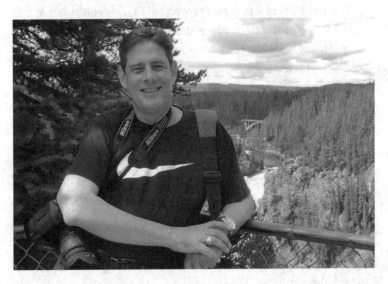

HAVE I BEEN A FOOL?

October 25, 2015

Most Christians don't like having their faith challenged. I'll admit to being one of them. I've always been more of a "let my walking do my talking" kind of guy. As I've said many times before, God and I have had many one-sided discussions about the purpose of the journey I'm on. The only time God has chosen to give me any type of an answer, it was, *They are watching*. He has yet to disclose to me who "they" are. I believe "they" are just people who know I'm a Christian and are watching to see how I respond to my journey and whether my faith still holds.

The reason this has come up in my mind is that I'm now fighting active lung cancer for the fourth time. We've been praying for complete healing for five years now. Instead of healing, we receive another diagnosis of recurring disease. I can't help but believe some of the people who are watching have to think I'm foolish to continue to believe there's a god who can or will heal me. After all, the psalms are full of passages where David's faith is ridiculed. Even Jesus was mocked while on the cross. Why should I be surprised if there are people questioning my faith in God?

To keep it real, I'll confess to having asked myself multiple times this past month if I was being foolish to believe God would heal me. There have been several nights I've stayed awake asking God where He is and imploring Him to show up. Yes, I freely admit to having fallen. One thing I've noticed in those times is that God isn't the one who has moved. It's always me who isn't where he's supposed to be. It's the times I've fallen that I find it easiest to worship God. I'm already down on my face before Him. Don't judge the absence of God by the times I've fallen, but judge the presence of God by the times that, thanks to His unfathomable grace, I've been able to stand.

Have I been a fool? I don't think so. In the Bible, we're instructed to work out our faith. In these last five years, I've come to believe that God allows trials to assist us in working out that faith. God doesn't mind the hard questions we ask. He expects them. While reading Psalm 37, I was reminded that my steps have been established by the Lord. Even when I fall, I won't be hurled headlong, because He's the One who is holding my hand.

I'm thankful that through this journey, what I believe has been transformed into faith.

A GOOD RIDE

June 25, 2016

Saturday morning was always my favorite time to go for a bike ride. I'd be up, dressed, and out the door before the first rays of sunshine began to peek over the horizon. There was just something about feeling the cool morning breeze on my face and pushing the pedals as the sun rose. Those mornings contain some of my favorite memories. I can remember where I was the first time I rode over thirty miles. The same for when I broke through the fifty-mile-ride limit. The first forty-five miles of that ride were a lot of fun. There was just something about pushing my body a little bit further than I thought it would go. On those mornings, as I rode home, I knew I'd had a good ride.

In many ways, this quest to beat lung cancer has been much the same. Many times I just had to push my body a little bit further than I thought it could go. The times I thought I couldn't make it any further, friends and family would lift us up. Sometimes they would come in person. Sometimes it was in their prayers. I've lost count of the times that DeLayne, the boys, and I have been blessed by the giving of others. Perhaps, the most surprising thing has been the many times we've been blessed by opportunities to give to other people. It's been a long journey that wouldn't have been possible without the help of others and the grace of God.

Yes, this journey has been a long one. There were twists and turns, never knowing what lay beyond the next bend in the road, but learning to trust that Jesus would be there waiting on us. It has taken us places we never thought we'd have to go, both physically and spiritually.

My earthly journey has come to an end. I now know what lay beyond the last bend in the road. I'm finally home resting in the loving arms of my Savior, Jesus Christ.

I've had a good ride.

DO NOT WORRY

by DeLayne Haga

"You worry too much." How many times had I heard that from Chris over the years?

Almost three weeks after Chris passed away, Shane mentioned he planned to make a leather wallet for himself, the craft his dad had taught him. Later, when I went upstairs to tell him good night, he was working on the design. In the bottom right corner, he had drawn a fancy 6 and a 25 with room for two more numbers.

"Thirty-four?" I asked.

"No—sixteen."

In memory of his dad, he was including the date of his dad's death on June 25, 2016.

Confused, he asked, "What made you think it would be the number thirty-four?"

"Matthew 6:25–34 was your dad's all-time favorite scripture. He asked that it be read at his funeral."

It was no accident I had walked in at that exact moment. Sometimes my thought processes are a little slow. It wasn't until the next morning I made the connection between June 25, the day Chris died, and his favorite Bible passage.

I hadn't understood why God prolonged the last day of Chris's life. God had a plan for His timetable. It wasn't a coincidence that Chris passed on Saturday, 6/25, at exactly 7:00 a.m. God knew all along that nothing else would give me such peace about my husband's passing as that date and precise time.

Even through his death, Chris was still reminding me, "Do not worry. God is in control."

"For this reason I say to you, do not be worried about your life, as to what you will eat or what you will drink; nor for your body, as to what you will put on. Is not life more than food, and the body more than clothing? Look at the birds of the air, that they do not sow, nor reap nor gather into barns, and yet your heavenly Father feeds them. Are you not worth much more than they? And who of you by being worried can add a single hour to his life? And why are you worried about clothing? Observe how the lilies of the field grow; they do not toil nor do they spin, yet I say to you that not even Solomon in all his glory clothed himself like one of these. But if God so clothes the grass of the field, which is alive today and tomorrow is thrown into the furnace, will He not much more clothe you? You of little faith! Do not worry then, saying, 'What will we eat?' or 'What will we drink?' or 'What will we wear for clothing?' For the Gentiles eagerly seek all these things; for your heavenly Father knows that you need all these things. But seek first His kingdom and His righteousness, and all these things will be added to you.

"So do not worry about tomorrow; for tomorrow will care for itself. Each day has enough trouble of its own."

—MATTHEW 6:25–34

THE LAST WORD

By DeLayne Haga

Cancer didn't have the last word—God did. As our friend Tom Wohlgamuth said at the graveside service, "Chris didn't lose his battle with cancer. Cancer lost its battle with Chris. When the cancer conquered his body, the cancer stopped living. It died. Forever. But Chris lives because Jesus conquered sin and death for us!"

> *"I am the resurrection and the life; he who believes in Me will live even if he dies, and everyone who lives and believes in Me will never die."*
>
> —JOHN 11:25

Chris gained victory over death. His spirit lives on and continues to help others in their battle and in their walk with the Lord as we share our story with you. I believe this verse answers my husband's long-sought-after purpose for having cancer.

> *"This sickness is not to end in death, but for the glory of God, so that the Son of God may be glorified by it."*
>
> —JOHN 11:4

After Chris was diagnosed with this terminal disease, we spent plenty of time in waiting rooms and hospitals with opportunities to think about the hand we'd been dealt. Cancer reminded us that life is precious, while giving us an opportunity to see God in many different ways.

Our relationship with the Lord deepened as we felt the depth of His outpouring love for us over and over again. We realized that even if Chris were to lose his battle against the cancer, we could find comfort knowing he would still have eternal life with the Lord. What greater love is there?

God deeply loves you. You don't believe it? Look at the cross. He loved His Son yet sacrificed Him to pay the penalty for our sins so that we would be able to spend eternity in heaven.

You may not have cancer, but your life is terminal. You just don't necessarily know what your cause of death will be or when your time will be up. Do you know, without a doubt, where you will spend eternity if you were to die today?

Have you accepted His love or rejected it? Can you imagine being a parent and having your child reject your love and shut you out of his life? Your grief wouldn't compare to the grief our heavenly Father must feel if you reject His free gift of eternal salvation.

"But I've lived a life full of sin. How could God love me?" you may ask.

There's no sin so big He won't forgive you. Denying Christ is the only thing that will prevent you from entering the kingdom of heaven. If you've never invited Jesus into your life but want to do so, simply pray something like this:

"Dear Lord, I admit I've sinned in my life and ask you to forgive me. I believe You're the Son of God and that You died on the cross to take the punishment for my sin. I believe You were buried and rose again from the grave. Thank You for Your gift of eternal life. I accept that gift and invite you into my life as my personal Savior. I choose to follow You into eternity. It's in Jesus' name I pray. Amen."

For the wages of sin is death, but the free gift of God is eternal life in Christ Jesus our Lord.

—ROMANS 6:23

AFTERWORD: PAYING HOMAGE

By Shane Haga

I can still remember my dad pulling out his leather tools to do some work on a wallet pattern at the kitchen table. I was maybe four or five years old and was excited to see what he was about to do. That night, he created a memory that would last a lifetime as he introduced me to leatherwork, patiently helping me as I clinched the swivel knife with my entire hand, trying to stay on the line.

As years passed, we both pulled the tools out of the closet to dabble here and there, only to stash them away once more.

A few years after being diagnosed with stage IV lung cancer, he dug the tools out of the closet in search of escape. It was then that I finally fell in love with the craft. Leatherwork created a new opportunity to bond with my dad, which I had been long-ing for since his treatment ruled out baseball and cycling. My dad helped me complete a wallet that year—the first functional leather piece I'd ever made.

In 2016 I decided to delve into the creative possibilities that leatherwork offers. I started with a journal, a Bible cover, and then a guitar strap. Requests began to roll in, and I sold my first piece. I had already exhausted my dad's knowledge of the craft, but every new project I started, I would, at some point, carry to him for approval.

On June 25, 2016, my dad's six-year battle with cancer came to an end, but I determined to carry on with the leatherwork.

After selling numerous pieces to friends and family, I decided to officially launch my own business, Homage Leatherworks. I remember my dad telling me he was offered the chance to sell belts at his local leather shop when he was younger, but he turned down the opportunity. When faced with the same decision, I chose to set up shop for the both of us.

With each custom piece I create, there comes a time when I think about showing him what I've made. Although it's a painful reminder that it's no longer an option, it also serves to remind me that a piece of my father lives on through me. I want to create not only beautiful leather goods, but pieces as meaningful to the buyer as they are to me, to be cherished forever.

This is my homage.

In memory of Chris Haga

www.homageleatherworks.com
www.facebook.com/homageleatherworks
www.instagram.com/homageleatherworks
https://twitter.com/HomageLW

APPENDIX: LUNG CANCER
STATISTICS AND SYMPTOMS

- Ten to fifteen percent of lung cancer cases are in never-smokers.
- Sixty to sixty-five percent of all new lung cancer diagnoses are among people who have never smoked or are former smokers.[1]

The signs and symptoms of lung cancer can take years to develop, and they may not appear until the disease is advanced. Some symptoms of lung cancer are in the chest:

- Coughing, especially if it persists or becomes intense
- Pain in the chest, shoulder, or back unrelated to pain from coughing
- A change in color or volume of sputum
- Shortness of breath
- Changes in the voice or being hoarse
- Harsh sounds with each breath
- Recurrent lung problems, such as bronchitis or pneumonia
- Coughing up phlegm or mucus, especially if it is tinged with blood
- Coughing up blood

---

[1] Source: www.lungevity.org

If the original lung cancer has spread, a person may feel symptoms in other places in the body. Common places for lung cancer to spread include other parts of the lungs, lymph nodes, bones, brain, liver, and adrenal glands. Some symptoms of lung cancer that may occur elsewhere in the body:

- Loss of appetite or unexplained weight loss
- Muscle wasting
- Fatigue
- Headaches, bone or joint pain
- Bone fractures not related to accidental injury
- Neurological symptoms, such as unsteady gait or memory loss
- Neck or facial swelling
- General weakness
- Bleeding
- Blood clots

Any unusual symptoms should be reported to your doctor.[2]

---

[2] Source: www.lungcancer.org

To see Chris's journey through the eyes of his caregiver
and to see how God worked in both their lives,
read DeLayne Haga's companion book:

His Love Carries Me
A Caregiver's Story of Faith, Hope, & Love

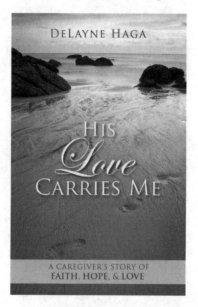

www.hagabooksoffaith.com
www.facebook.com/hagabooksoffaith
https://twitter.com/hagabooksfaith

ABOUT THE AUTHOR

Chris Haga earned a Bachelor of Science in Electronics Engineering Technology from Oklahoma State University with a Master of Business Administration from the University of Dallas. He worked thirty-one years for Texas Instruments as an engineer and was working full time until just two weeks prior to his death.

A devoted husband and father, Chris and his wife, DeLayne, were married for thirty-two years and raised two sons. Besides cycling, he enjoyed photographing nature and doing leather-craft work.

Chris loved riding his bike for exercise and was riding eighty miles a week when diagnosed with stage IV lung cancer that had metastasized to his brain. *He had never smoked.*

The mass in his lungs grew to 13 centimeters before doctors found a successful regimen to shrink it. He was given six months to live, but he lived six *years* and achieved "no evidence of disease" on three separate occasions. He continued riding his bike another four years despite cancer and only having one good lung.

Chris participated in four clinical trials, helping to advance medical science to fight lung cancer. The FDA approved two of the drugs while he was in the trials. One groundbreaking study that he donated blood for is now enabling doctors to identify some lung cancers by using liquid biopsies instead of invasive surgical procedures.

He was a devout Christian and became a regular at his church's Cancer Encouragement Group. He mentored other lung cancer survivors and worked to raise public awareness that people who have never smoked can get lung cancer.

Chris desperately wanted something good to come from his cancer experience that would help others and to glorify the Lord through his life. He succeeded in both.

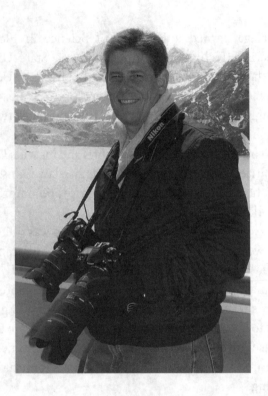